Level I Practice Exams – Vc

SCHWESER 2013 CFA LEVEL I PRACTICE EXAMS VOLUME 2

Published in 2012 by Kaplan Schweser.
Printed in the United States of America.
ISBN: 978-1-4277-4225-4 / 1-4277-4225-1
PPN: 3200-2865

Use Your Schweser Online Access Account

All purchasers of this book are sent login information for Online Access in an e-mail. This is your login to use Performance Tracker and access other Schweser online resources. Simply log in at www.schweser.com and select "Online Access" to use any of these features. If you need password help, go to www.schweser.com/password or use the "Password Help" link that appears if your login is unsuccessful.

Volume 2 Online Features at a Glance

Links to Curriculum

Within the online answer explanations, we have included page references to the relevant text in both the SchweserNotes and the CFA Institute program texts as well as the primary Learning Outcome Statement supporting the question.

Exam Diagnostics

When you enter your answers in our Performance Tracker utility, you can request a breakdown of your overall score on any one-half (120 question) exam. See how you performed by topic area, study session, or reading. You can also get the Learning Outcome Statement references for just those questions you answered incorrectly to help you focus your review efforts.

Performance Comparison

When you enter your answers on the page for Performance Tracker, you can find out how your score on each half-exam compares to the scores of others who entered their answers.

Log in today and enjoy the benefits of Performance Tracker and the other online resources in your account.

How to Use This Book

Practice Exams are a very important part of the Schweser Study Program. **Don't neglect them.**

You shouldn't take the Level I CFA® Exam without lots of practice answering exam-like questions.

Test yourself with these Practice Exams only after you have completed all the assigned readings. As on the actual CFA exam, assume International Financial Reporting Standards (IFRS) apply unless a question indicates otherwise.

The purpose of these questions is to make sure that you know all the concepts and ideas that are in the assigned readings. If you truly know the material you will do well on the actual exam. While our practice questions cover all the material, **they are not actual exam questions.** Our practice exams are not designed to predict your score on the actual CFA exam, although we try to match the level of difficulty on the exam. Use them to practice and identify those areas in which you need additional work.

Remember though, that CFA Institute® tries very hard every year to come up with new and innovative ways to test you. Your only defense against a good exam writer is to actually know the material. Learning the material and how to pace yourself on the exam is what our practice questions are designed to help you do.

The CFA exam is structured so that the morning and afternoon exams are each independent exams covering all topic areas. So, the three 6-hour practice exams here in Volume 2 really are six 3-hour practice exams. This gives you several opportunities to test your progress.

Our recommendations for using this book are:

- After you have finished your first complete review of the assigned reading material, take the morning portion of Practice Exam 1, paying strict attention to the time constraint. Enter your answers online. Performance Tracker will identify your weak spots and point you toward the material you need to review. Go back and study the material related to your weak areas.
- After you have reviewed that material, take the afternoon portion of Practice Exam 1. Again, pay strict attention to the allotted time and review the material related to your weak areas identified by Performance Tracker.
- During the weeks prior to the exam, set aside two days to take Exams 2 and 3. Complete each of these 6-hour exams on one day with only a lunch break between the two halves. This will get you used to doing what you must do on exam day. Again review your weak areas but also look at the explanation for every problem you missed, so it won't happen again.
- Finally, review all of Study Session 1 on the day before the exam. Ethical and Professional Standards and Global Investment Performance Standards will be approximately 15% of the Level I exam. A final review of this material, including all the text and all the examples in the *Standards of Practice Handbook,* will serve you well on exam day.

Don't plan on passing the exam by memorizing questions and answers. Instead, learn the reasoning behind each of the questions. CFA Institute® isn't going to ask you our questions, but they will ask you questions that address the same concepts, logic, and definitions necessary to answer the practice exam questions.

Exam 1
Morning Session

Topic	Questions	Points
Ethical and Professional Standards	1–18	27
Quantitative Methods	19–32	21
Economics	33–44	18
Financial Reporting and Analysis	45–68	36
Corporate Finance	69–78	15
Portfolio Management	79–84	9
Equity Investments	85–96	18
Fixed Income	97–110	21
Derivatives	111–116	9
Alternative Investments	117–120	6
Total		**180**

Test Answers

1. A B C
2. A B C
3. A B C
4. A B C
5. A B C
6. A B C
7. A B C
8. A B C
9. A B C
10. A B C
11. A B C
12. A B C
13. A B C
14. A B C
15. A B C
16. A B C
17. A B C
18. A B C
19. A B C
20. A B C
21. A B C
22. A B C
23. A B C
24. A B C
25. A B C
26. A B C
27. A B C
28. A B C
29. A B C
30. A B C
31. A B C
32. A B C
33. A B C
34. A B C
35. A B C
36. A B C
37. A B C
38. A B C
39. A B C
40. A B C
41. A B C
42. A B C
43. A B C
44. A B C
45. A B C
46. A B C
47. A B C
48. A B C
49. A B C
50. A B C
51. A B C
52. A B C
53. A B C
54. A B C
55. A B C
56. A B C
57. A B C
58. A B C
59. A B C
60. A B C
61. A B C
62. A B C
63. A B C
64. A B C
65. A B C
66. A B C
67. A B C
68. A B C
69. A B C
70. A B C
71. A B C
72. A B C
73. A B C
74. A B C
75. A B C
76. A B C
77. A B C
78. A B C
79. A B C
80. A B C
81. A B C
82. A B C
83. A B C
84. A B C
85. A B C
86. A B C
87. A B C
88. A B C
89. A B C
90. A B C
91. A B C
92. A B C
93. A B C
94. A B C
95. A B C
96. A B C
97. A B C
98. A B C
99. A B C
100. A B C
101. A B C
102. A B C
103. A B C
104. A B C
105. A B C
106. A B C
107. A B C
108. A B C
109. A B C
110. A B C
111. A B C
112. A B C
113. A B C
114. A B C
115. A B C
116. A B C
117. A B C
118. A B C
119. A B C
120. A B C

Exam 1
Morning Session

Questions 1 through 18 relate to Ethical and Professional Standards. (27 minutes)

1. Ed Socho states that in a GIPS-compliant presentation, (1) total firm value must be based on the market values of all accounts including non-fee-paying accounts and accounts where the client makes the investment decisions, and that (2) the firm must include the performance results of third-party advisors selected by the firm in composite performance. Are Socho's statements accurate?
   A. Both of these statements are accurate.
   B. Neither of these statements is accurate.
   C. Only one of these statements is accurate.

2. Upon completing investment reports on equity securities, Shannon Mason, CFA, routinely shreds all documents used in preparing the reports. In a report on UltraTech Software, Mason provides detailed explanations of the upside and downside risks associated with UltraTech, but provides no information on a sharp decrease in insider buying over the last 12 months. Mason has *most likely* violated:
   A. CFA Institute Standards by failing to maintain adequate records.
   B. CFA Institute Standards by neglecting to include the insider buying information in the investment report.
   C. none of the Standards.

3. William Callahan, CFA, is an energy analyst. His supervisor, Nancy Deininger, CFA, has recently decided to let Callahan cover a few of the firms that Deininger had been covering previously. Deininger gives Callahan specific instructions not to change her prior recommendation on one of these firms, Mayfield Energy. Callahan's *least* appropriate action is to:
   A. tell Deininger that he cannot cover Mayfield Energy under those restrictions.
   B. perform his own independent analysis of Mayfield and reach an independent conclusion.
   C. use ambiguous language in the report, in order to not mislead the investor while complying with his employer's instructions.

4. Wayne Sergeant, CFA, is an independent investment advisor who works with individuals. A longtime client asks Sergeant if he can recommend an attorney. Sergeant refers his client to Jim Chapman, a local attorney who is also a friend of Sergeant's. Previously, Chapman had agreed to perform some legal work for Sergeant in exchange for the referral of new clients. Do Sergeant's actions violate CFA Institute Standards of Professional Conduct?
   A. No, because the client is under no obligation and is still free to select another attorney.
   B. Yes, because Sergeant is prohibited from a making recommendations that could be considered biased due to his friendship with Chapman.
   C. Yes, because Sergeant did not disclose the nature of his arrangement with Chapman to his client.

5. Linda Schultz, CFA, is an investment advisor at Wheaton Investments. Schultz has been employed there for five years, and has never signed a "non-compete" clause. While at Wheaton, Schultz makes preparations to set up her own money management firm. She does not contact any existing clients before leaving Wheaton and does not take any firm records or files. After her resignation becomes effective, Schultz replicates a list of former clients from memory and uses public sources to get their contact information. She then contacts these former clients and solicits their business for her new firm. Has Schultz violated any CFA Institute Standards?
   A. Yes. Schultz may not contact clients of her old firm.
   B. No. Schultz is in compliance with CFA Institute Standards.
   C. Yes. Schultz is permitted to notify clients that she has left her old firm, but she cannot encourage them to come with her to the new firm.

6. Recommended procedures for compliance with the Standard concerning misconduct suggest that firms in the investment industry should:
   A. periodically test their employees' knowledge of applicable laws, regulations, and the firm's code of ethics.
   B. periodically inform employees of violations that have occurred and the disciplinary actions that the firm took against the employees involved.
   C. check references of potential employees to verify that they are of good character and eligible for employment in the investment industry.

7. Darlene Hess, CFA, manages a pension fund that has a sizeable position in Knoll Corporation common stock. Hess also holds Knoll common stock in her personal account. Hess participates in an analyst conference call in which Knoll's chief financial officer advises that the company's current-quarter earnings will slip below consensus forecast. Knoll has not disclosed this to the public. Hess believes news of the poor earnings will reduce the stock's value significantly. Hess may:
   A. not sell Knoll stock from either the pension fund or her personal account.
   B. sell Knoll stock from her personal account but may not sell it from the pension fund.
   C. sell Knoll stock from the pension fund but may not sell it from her personal account.

8. Sue Seros, CFA, is reviewing the performance of Arithmatics, Inc., which she has placed in several client accounts. She believes a recent decrease in its price may present a buying opportunity and that industry conditions suggest Arithmatics may be an attractive acquisition for a larger company. She has occasion to talk to her podiatrist, who mentions Arithmatics and tells her that he believes Arithmatics is a takeover target and that she should buy more. Seros subsequently increases her clients' holdings in Arithmatics and tells her clients that it is an attractive takeover prospect at current prices. Seros has:
   A. not violated the Standards of Practice.
   B. violated the Standard on material nonpublic information.
   C. violated the Standard on diligence and reasonable basis.

9 The Code and Standards prohibit a Member or Candidate who has left one employer and joined another from:
   A. soliciting the old employer's clients.
   B. misappropriating client lists.
   C. transferring files from the old employer to the new employer.

10. Juan Perez, CFA, is an airline industry analyst. Perez does not currently cover New Jet, a relatively new airline. New Jet believes its new service is unique and has offered two first class tickets to research analysts in the hopes of receiving increased coverage. Perez believes he can more fully understand the airline's new concept if he is a passenger, so he accepts the tickets and takes his girlfriend on a weekend trip. Perez does not see any differentiation between New Jet and other airlines, and decides the company is too small to warrant analytical coverage. According to the Code and Standards, Perez:
A. was required to reject the offer of the airline tickets from New Jet.
B. should have obtained written permission from his employer before accepting the airline tickets.
C. did not need written permission from his employer before accepting the tickets because the offer did not conflict with his employer's interests.

11. When regulations in a GIPS-compliant firm's home country conflict with GIPS, the firm must:
A. present results in compliance with GIPS, and must separately present results following country-specific regulations.
B. follow any applicable country-specific regulations and disclose the conflict in the GIPS-compliant presentation.
C. disclose the nature of the conflict with GIPS-mandated presentation results to the regulatory body associated with the country in which there is a conflict.

12. Jon Jamerson, CFA, is an investment analyst. Alco, Inc. offers Jamerson a small number of shares in Alco's oversubscribed IPO. Is Jamerson violating CFA Institute Standards by accepting these shares for his personal account?
A. Accepting these shares does not violate the Code and Standards.
B. Jamerson has violated the Standard concerning independence and objectivity.
C. Jamerson has violated the Standard governing conduct as Members and Candidates in the CFA Program.

13. Peter Kent, CFA, is an investment manager. Kent just accepted a new client, Lois Parker, who is of the same approximate age, income bracket, and net worth as Kent's other clients. Kent therefore decides to invest Parker's funds according to a model that he uses for his clients that efficiently diversifies funds across all industries. Parker agrees to Kent's investment plan since she has no prior investment experience and prefers to let an expert manage her money. With respect to suitability, Kent has:
A. complied with the Standards since the client agreed to the strategy.
B. violated the Standards by failing to determine Parker's investment objectives and constraints.
C. violated the Standards by failing to provide a thorough description of the model used to invest the funds.

14. Bob Reynolds, CFA, is bearish on JBH Manufacturing Company and takes a short position in the stock. Reynolds posts negative claims about company management, which are untrue, to several popular investment bulletin boards on the Internet. According to CFA Institute Standards of Professional Conduct, Reynolds has violated the Standard concerning:
A. fair dealing.
B. communication with clients.
C. market manipulation.

15. Judy Nicely, CFA, works for a large brokerage firm managing portfolios for individuals. In a meeting with Patty Owen, a client, Nicely suggests moving a portion of Owen's portfolio to U.S. bank certificates of deposit. Nicely states that the principal is guaranteed up to Federal Deposit Insurance Corporation limits. Nicely has:
A. complied with CFA Institute Standards.
B. violated the Standards by making an inappropriate assurance or guarantee.
C. violated the Standards by misrepresenting the terms and character of the investment.

16. The Standard on performance presentation *least likely* recommends that Members and Candidates:
A. disclose whether performance is gross or net of fees.
B. support any forecast of future performance with actual data on past performance.
C. include terminated accounts in performance history.

17. To comply with the Standard on material nonpublic information, is it permissible for a research analyst for a large, multiservice firm, who has responsibility for issuing investment recommendations on a company, to assist the investment banking side during a transaction with that company?
    A. This is never permitted under CFA Institute Standards.
    B. The Member or Candidate may provide limited assistance under tight controls.
    C. This would be allowed only if the Member or Candidate is making a permanent move to the investment banking side of the firm.

18. Joe Howard, CFA, is responsible for reviewing an investment firm's promotional materials before they are released to the public. Howard finds these two statements:

    Statement 1: "As a CFA charterholder, Mel Buckmaster is a highly qualified financial manager who will achieve superior investment returns."

    Statement 2: "Tom Waters, C.F.A., has been promoted to Senior Portfolio Analyst."

    Do these statements comply with the Code and Standards?
    A. Both of these statements comply with the Code and Standards.
    B. Neither of these statements complies with the Code and Standards.
    C. Only one of these statements complies with the Code and Standards.

Questions 19 through 32 relate to Quantitative Methods. (21 minutes)

19. The probability that quarterly earnings for Phone Buddies, Inc. will increase in any quarter is 75%, and the probability that its quarterly earnings will decrease is 25%. The probability that Phone Buddies earnings will increase in any five of the next eight quarters is between:
    A. 0 and 5%.
    B. 5% and 15%.
    C. 15% and 25%.

20. A recent study indicates that the probability that a company's earnings will exceed consensus expectations equals 50%. From this analysis, the odds that the company's earnings exceed expectations are:
    A. 1 to 2.
    B. 2 to 1.
    C. 1 to 1.

21. Mervin Erikson, CFA, is the portfolio manager of a large capitalization mutual fund. Erikson uses the S&P 500 index fund as his benchmark. Erikson provides the following 10-year data:

- The annual excess return of the large capitalization mutual fund is 8.3%.
- The annual standard deviation of the large capitalization mutual fund is 43%.
- The S&P 500 index fund generated a return of 7.9%.
- The S&P 500 index fund has an annual standard deviation of 26%.
- The annual risk-free rate is 3.0%.

On a risk-adjusted basis:
A. the S&P 500 index fund had superior performance.
B. the large capitalization mutual fund had superior performance.
C. the S&P 500 index fund and the large capitalization mutual fund had the same performance.

22. An analyst believes that two variables, X and Y, are both normally distributed. To test the hypotheses that the variance of X is equal to 7 and that the variance of X is equal to the variance of Y, he should use, respectively, a(n):

	Var(X) = 7	Var(X) = Var(Y)
A.	Chi square test	*F*-test
B.	Chi square test	Chi square test
C.	*F*-test	Chi square test

23. Tracking error is *most accurately* described as the difference between:
A. a sample mean and the mean of the distribution.
B. a moving average of closing prices and the most recent closing price.
C. the total return on a portfolio and the total return on its benchmark index.

24. When estimating a population mean or constructing a confidence interval based on the central limit theorem:
A. the midpoint of a confidence interval is a point estimate of the population parameter.
B. the degree of significance is the probability that the actual value of the parameter lies within the confidence interval.
C. a point estimate with a 95% degree of confidence is more accurate than a point estimate with a 90% degree of confidence.

25. Pat Harris, CFA, examines earnings data for 3 energy companies:

Company	Average per-share quarterly earnings	*p*-value
Axxon Industries	$2.00	0.25
Babson Drilling	$0.50	0.04
Cerex Energy	$3.00	0.01

Harris is asked to test the hypothesis for each company that mean earnings equal zero. Using a 5% level of significance, Harris should conclude that the null hypothesis should be rejected for:

A. Babson only.
B. Axxon and Cerex only.
C. Babson and Cerex only.

26. Analyst Shelly King is using a returns and earnings database to examine the past performance of stocks. King sorts stocks from high to low P/E ratio by dividing the beginning of the year stock price by the reported year-end earnings per share recorded in the database for the prior year. King then creates portfolios of high P/E stocks and low P/E stocks and compares their performance. King's research design *most likely* suffers from:

A. time period bias.
B. data mining bias.
C. look-ahead bias.

27. Don Faust, CFA, is reviewing Metro Utility Corporation. Based on historical data, Metro increases its dividend 80% of the time given rising GDP and 30% of the time given falling GDP. Faust believes that there is a 30% probability that GDP will decrease. The probability that Metro will increase its dividend and GDP will increase is *closest* to:

A. 14%.
B. 24%.
C. 56%.

28. Cheryl Smith, CFA, conducts a study comparing dividend changes for energy and non-energy companies. Smith determines that 15% of the stock market universe consists of energy companies. Smith also determines that the probability that an energy company will increase its dividend is 90% and the probability that a non-energy company will increase its dividend is 30%. After conducting her analysis, Smith randomly selects one company from the universe of stocks from the most recent quarter and notices that the company declared a dividend increase. The probability that Smith randomly selected an energy company is *closest* to:

A. 5%.
B. 15%.
C. 35%.

29. Jane Wilcott, CFA, is researching whether value stocks can be expected to outperform growth stocks in any given month. Examining 10 years of monthly returns on a value stock portfolio and a growth stock portfolio, Wilcott records a positive sign for any month the return on the value portfolio exceeded that of the growth portfolio, and a negative sign for any month the return on the value portfolio was less than that of the growth portfolio. Wilcott tests the null hypothesis that the number of positive months is less than or equal to the number of negative months. Wilcott's research design is an example of a:
A. binomial test.
B. conditional test.
C. nonparametric test.

30. The probability of a good economy is 0.55 and the probability of a poor economy is 0.45. Given a good economy, the probability that the earnings of HomeBuilder Inc. will increase is 0.60 and the probability that earnings will not increase is 0.40. Given a poor economy, the probability that earnings will increase is 0.30 and the probability that earnings will not increase is 0.70. The unconditional probability of an increase in earnings is *closest* to:
A. 0.18.
B. 0.47.
C. 0.90.

31. A sample of 250 observations has the following properties:

Mean	8.6
Standard deviation	4.9
Sample kurtosis	3.0
Median	8.3
Mode	8.1

This sample *most likely* has:
A. at least one observation equal to 8.3.
B. sample skewness greater than zero.
C. positive excess kurtosis.

32. Jessica Turner, CFA, is a financial analyst with Jet Inc. She is evaluating an investment project with the cash flows shown in the table below. Jet's cost of capital is 8%.

Year	*0*	*1*	*2*
Cash flow	($15,000)	$15,000	$15,000

The internal rate of return for the project is *closest* to:
A. 41%.
B. 62%.
C. 100%.

Questions 33 through 44 relate to Economics. (18 minutes)

33. In the short run, a perfectly competitive firm's supply curve is:
    A. upward sloping and its demand curve is perfectly elastic.
    B. upward sloping and its demand curve is downward sloping.
    C. perfectly inelastic and its demand curve is perfectly elastic.

34. Other things equal, aggregate demand is *most likely* to decrease as a result of a decrease in:
    A. taxes.
    B. the money supply.
    C. the foreign exchange value of the domestic currency.

35. Which of the following *most likely* describes a loss that consumers suffer under an unregulated monopoly compared to a competitive market?
    A. Monopolies produce less goods than a competitive market would.
    B. Costs of production are higher with monopolies.
    C. Monopolists charge the maximum price.

36. Setting a minimum wage above the equilibrium wage:
    A. results in increased unemployment, and setting a minimum wage below the equilibrium wage has no effect on unemployment.
    B. has no effect on unemployment, and setting a minimum wage below the equilibrium wage results in increased unemployment.
    C. results in increased unemployment, and setting a minimum wage below the equilibrium minimum wage results in decreased unemployment.

37. Consider two currencies, the VKN and the PKR. The PKR is trading at a one-year forward premium relative to the VKN of 2.3%. The one-year riskless PKR rate is 3.0%. If no arbitrage opportunities are available, the current one-year riskless VKN rate is *closest* to:
    A. 0.7%.
    B. 2.3%.
    C. 5.3%.

38. Which of the following statements about models of international trade is *least accurate*?
    A. The Ricardian model of trade uses labor as the only factor of production.
    B. The Heckscher-Ohlin model asserts that the source of competitive advantage is differences in the relative amounts of labor and capital a country possesses.
    C. Considering both labor and capital as factors of production, the price of the more available factor of production will decrease.

39. Pauker Company is producing at minimum short-run marginal cost. Pauker is *most likely* also producing:
    A. maximum profits.
    B. at maximum marginal product.
    C. at minimum average variable cost.

40. Which of the following amounts is *least likely* to be subtracted from gross domestic product in order to calculate national income?
    A. Statistical discrepancy.
    B. Indirect business taxes.
    C. Capital consumption allowance.

41. The kinked demand curve oligopoly model is based on a belief that:
    A. competing firms that collude to restrict output each have an incentive to cheat.
    B. a firm's competitors will follow a price decrease but will not follow a price increase.
    C. a firm can increase profits by charging different prices to distinct groups of consumers.

42. If a market has a supply curve that intersects the demand curve from above, a price below equilibrium will lead to:
    A. excess supply that will tend to decrease the price.
    B. excess demand that will tend to increase the price.
    C. excess demand that will tend to decrease the price.

43. An analyst who expects the economy to experience stagflation should *most appropriately* recommend investing in:
    A. bonds.
    B. equities.
    C. commodities.

44. If the inflation rate is higher than the central bank's target rate, an appropriate monetary policy response is to:
    A. decrease the required reserve ratio.
    B. increase the interest rate for borrowed reserves.
    C. purchase government securities in the open market.

Questions 45 through 68 relate to Financial Reporting and Analysis. (36 minutes)

45. The choice of perpetual versus periodic inventory system is *most likely* to result in different values for gross profit when the inventory valuation method used is:
    A. last in, first out.
    B. first in, first out.
    C. specific identification.

46. Accrued revenue is shown on the balance sheet as:
    A. an asset.
    B. a liability.
    C. owners' equity.

47. Sam Jones, CFA, is analyzing a company whose financial information provides reconciliation between net income reported under U.S. GAAP and net income reported under IFRS. Jones states the following:

    Statement 1: IFRS require three years of comparative financial information, while U.S. GAAP has no specific requirement.

    Statement 2: Both IFRS and U.S. GAAP permit the use of extraordinary items.

    Is Jones correct with respect to these statements?
    A. Both of these statements are correct.
    B. Neither of these statements is correct.
    C. Only one of these statements is correct.

48. Kimble Corporation does not record an estimate for the amount of revenues that may be uncollectible. What effect will this omission have on the company's financial statements?
    A. Overstate assets.
    B. Overstate liabilities.
    C. Understate net income.

49. In which step of the financial statement analysis framework should an analyst create adjusted financial statements?
    A. Collect data.
    B. Process data.
    C. Analyze and interpret data.

50. Roome Corp. has 5,000,000 common shares outstanding. There are 500,000 warrants outstanding to purchase the stock at $20, and there are 200,000 options outstanding to buy the stock at $50. The average market price for the stock over the year was $40, and the current stock price is $60. The number of shares used to calculate diluted EPS is:
    A. 5,250,000 shares.
    B. 5,300,000 shares.
    C. 5,700,000 shares.

51. Tom Carter, CFA, is analyzing Sydex Company. Sydex is capitalizing interest costs on its long-lived assets. Carter adjusts Sydex's financials to treat the capitalized interest costs for the most recent period as an expense. After Carter's adjustments, Sydex's interest coverage ratio will be:
    A. lower.
    B. higher.
    C. unaffected.

52. An investor has obtained the following information about Worldwide Industries, Inc.

Net profit margin	8.7%
Total asset turnover	2.4 times
Dividend payout ratio	35%
Tax rate	35%
Total sales	$120 million
Total equity	40% of total assets

    Based on this information, Worldwide's ROE is *closest* to:
    A. 8.4%.
    B. 20.0%.
    C. 52.2%.

53. Both IFRS and U.S. GAAP allow deferred taxes to be:
    A. presented as noncurrent on the balance sheet.
    B. measured using a substantially enacted tax rate.
    C. recognized in equity after a fixed asset revaluation.

54. Which of the following *most* accurately describes cash flow classification under U.S. GAAP and IFRS?
    A. Dividends paid are a financing activity under U.S. GAAP and dividends received may be shown as an operating or investing activity under IFRS.
    B. Dividends received may be shown as an operating or investing activity under U.S. GAAP and dividends paid is a financing activity under IFRS.
    C. Interest expense is a financing activity under U.S. GAAP and interest received may be shown as an operating or investing activity under IFRS.

55. An accountant with Umble Company is preparing the statement of cash flows. Cash flow from operations is $210 and cash on the balance sheet increased by $340. Transactions during the period include:

Capital expenditures	$100
Investment in joint venture	40
Acquisitions	80
Dividends from affiliates	25

Umble's cash flow from financing (CFF) under U.S. GAAP is:
A. –$220.
B. +$195.
C. +$350.

56. Forman Inc. and Swoft Inc. both operate within the same industry. Forman's stated strategy is to differentiate its premium products relative to its competitors, while Swoft is a low-cost producer. Given the companies' stated strategies, Forman *most likely* has:
A. higher gross margins relative to Swoft.
B. lower advertising expenses relative to Swoft.
C. lower research and development expenses relative to Swoft.

57. Skinner Inc. manufactures and sells kitchen utensils. Over time, the cost of Skinner's inventory has been rising. A recent jump in demand for Skinner's products has resulted in a LIFO liquidation. What effect, if any, will the LIFO liquidation have on Skinner's gross profit margin percentage?
A. Increase.
B. Decrease.
C. No effect.

58. Inventory cost is *most likely* to include:
A. storage costs for finished goods until they are actually sold.
B. shipping cost for delivery to the customer.
C. an allocation of fixed production overhead.

59. For a firm that reports its long-term debt at market value, a decrease in the rating on its long-term debt will:
A. decrease its debt-to-assets ratio.
B. decrease its equity.
C. have no effect on its reported solvency ratios.

60. Dubois Company bought land five years ago for €2 million and presents its balance sheet value as €2.2 million. If the fair value of the land decreases to €1.8 million, Dubois will *most likely*:
   A. decrease shareholders' equity by €400,000 but will not recognize a loss.
   B. recognize a loss of €200,000 and decrease shareholders' equity by €400,000.
   C. recognize a loss of €400,000 and decrease shareholders' equity by €200,000.

61. Royt Corp. has experienced a 2-year period of depressed operating results. This has led Royt's management to look for ways to show more favorable operating cash flow without violating International Financial Reporting Standards. A strategy that is *most likely* to help meet this goal is:
   A. reducing days' sales in payables.
   B. securitizing accounts receivable.
   C. recognizing impairment of long-lived assets.

62. Pickett Company reports on its financial statements for 20X9:
   - 20X9 taxable income = $5,000.
   - Deferred tax asset year-end 20X8 = $2,000.
   - Deferred tax liability year-end 20X8 = $1,000.
   - 20X9 temporary differences creating deferred tax liabilities = $600.
   - 20X9 temporary differences creating deferred tax assets = $200.

   In 20X9, the tax rate increases from 35% to 50%. Pickett's income tax expense for 20X9 is *closest* to:

   A. $2,300.
   B. $2,500.
   C. $2,700.

63. Topper Company's sales for December are $3 million. Cash received in December from these sales is $1 million. Under accrual accounting, the $2 million difference will be reported on Topper's financial statements as:
   A. accrued revenue.
   B. unearned revenue.
   C. an accrued liability.

64. Harter Corporation issued $95 million of 10-year 8% coupon bonds in 20X5. In 20X5, the market interest rate was 6%. The current market interest rate is 9%. Harter has generated unexpectedly strong profits over the last several years. Given a high cash balance, the company is considering repurchasing the entire bond issue. If Harter repurchases the bonds, what is the immediate effect in Harter's income statement?
A. A loss is recognized.
B. A gain is recognized.
C. No gain or loss is recognized.

65. An analyst creates a common-size cash flow statement for Wheelan Company:

Wheelan Co. Cash Flow Statement (Percent of revenues)

	20X8	*20X9*
Net income	6.6%	5.8%
Depreciation	2.6%	3.0%
Inventory	0.2%	0.3%
Accrued liabilities	0.2%	–0.2%
Cash from operating activities	**9.6%**	**9.0%**
Plant and equipment	–8.0%	–8.3%
Other investing cash flows	0.1%	–0.2%
Cash from investing activities	**–7.9%**	**–8.5%**
Cash dividends paid	–0.5%	–0.8%
Issuance (retirement) of stock, net	–3.3%	–2.4%
Issuance (retirement) of debt, net	3.1%	4.6%
Cash from financing activities	**–0.8%**	**1.4%**
Total cash flow	**0.9%**	**1.9%**

The common-size cash flow statement *most likely* suggests that Wheelan's:
A. net income is decreasing.
B. cash flow to revenue ratio is decreasing.
C. investment in plant and equipment is decreasing.

66. Varin, Inc. purchases franchise rights with an estimated useful life of ten years and a trademark that can be renewed every five years for a nominal fee. Under IFRS, Varin will recognize amortization expense on:
A. both of these assets.
B. neither of these assets.
C. only one of these assets.

67. If the quick ratio is equal to 2.0, a decrease in inventory and an equal decrease in accounts payable will:
A. increase the quick ratio.
B. decrease the quick ratio.
C. leave the quick ratio unchanged.

68. Under U.S. GAAP, the expected return on plan assets for a defined benefit pension plan is reported as:
A. net income in the current period.
B. other comprehensive income and is not amortized to income.
C. other comprehensive income and is amortized over time to income.

Questions 69 through 78 relate to Corporate Finance. (15 minutes)

69. Yang Yu is a board member for Broadcast Radio Group. Yu should *most likely* be considered an independent board member if he:
A. is a consultant to a subsidiary of Broadcast Radio Group.
B. serves on the board of directors for Broadcast Radio Group's auditors.
C. owns a significant non-controlling stock position in Broadcast Radio Group.

70. Isaac Segovia, CFA, is using the net present value (NPV) and internal rate of return (IRR) methods to analyze a project for his firm. After its initial cash outflow, the project will generate several years of cash inflows, but will require a net cash outflow in the final year. The problem Segovia is *most likely* to encounter when using the NPV or IRR methods for this analysis is:
A. multiple IRRs.
B. negative NPV.
C. conflicting NPV and IRR project rankings.

71. Shawn Wright, CFA, is evaluating the short-term investment policy for Hegeman Industries. Wright should *most likely* conclude that Hegeman's investment policy is:
A. inappropriate if it restricts the types of securities that can be held.
B. appropriate if it lists specific issuers from which Hegeman may purchase securities.
C. appropriate if it limits the proportion of the total portfolio that can be held in various types of issues.

72. QuaryCo is determining whether to expand its current production capacity. A feasibility study completed one year ago indicates that the rock in the new quarry site is of sufficient quality. The project would require an increase in working capital and the use of an empty factory owned by the company. Several existing customers would be expected to purchase materials from the new quarry due to its closer proximity. In evaluating the expansion project, QuaryCo should *least* appropriately consider:
A. cash expended to perform the feasibility study.
B. the increase in working capital required to support the project.
C. the effects of customers who will switch purchases to the new quarry.

73. Reviewing the performance and independence of board members is a responsibility of the:
A. audit committee.
B. nominations committee.
C. compensation committee.

74. Janet Adams, CFA, is reviewing Rival Company's financial statements. Rival's long-term debt totals $35 million, while total shareholder equity equals $140 million. Rival's long-term debt has a YTM of 9%. Rival's tax rate is 40% and its beta is 0.9. Adams gathers the following additional facts:

- Treasury bills earn 4.0%.
- The equity risk premium is 4.5%.

Based on the information provided, Rival's weighted average cost of capital is *closest* to:
A. 4.6%.
B. 7.5%.
C. 8.2%.

75. James Waverly, CFA, is discussing the use of marginal cost of capital as a discount rate for new projects and makes the following statements:

Statement 1: Marginal cost of capital is an appropriate discount rate for average-risk projects, but it should be adjusted for projects that are more risky or less risky than the average of current projects.

Statement 2: Using the marginal cost of capital as a discount rate assumes that the capital structure will remain constant over the life of the project being evaluated.

Are Waverly's statements accurate?
A. Both of these statements are accurate.
B. Neither of these statements is accurate.
C. Only one of these statements is accurate.

76. In reviewing the effectiveness of a company's working capital management, an analyst has calculated operating cycle and cash conversion cycle measures for the past three years.

	20X6	*20X7*	*20X8*
Operating cycle (number of days)	55	60	62
Cash conversion cycle (number of days)	27	30	32

The trends in the operating cycle and cash conversion cycle *most likely* indicate:
A. improving liquidity.
B. slower collections of receivables.
C. stretching of payables.

77. The following data are reported for Moving Vans, Inc.:

Dividend yield	5%
Dividend payout	20%
Return on equity	15%

Assuming Moving Vans' dividend yield, dividend payout, and return on equity will remain constant indefinitely, the cost of equity capital is *closest* to:
A. 15%.
B. 17%.
C. 19%.

78. A single independent project with a negative net present value has an initial cost of $2.5 million and would generate cash inflows of $1 million in each of the next three years. The discount rate the company used when evaluating this project is *closest* to:
A. 8%.
B. 9%.
C. 10%.

Questions 79 through 84 relate to Portfolio Management. (9 minutes)

79. Two stocks, Shaw Inc., and Melon Inc., have identical total risk. The Shaw stock risk is comprised of 60% systematic risk and 40% unsystematic risk, while the Melon stock risk is comprised of 40% systematic risk and 60% unsystematic risk. In equilibrium, according to capital market theory, Shaw has:
A. a higher expected return than Melon.
B. a lower expected return than Melon.
C. the same expected return as Melon.

80. If Investor 1 has steeper indifference curves for return as a function of risk than Investor 2, then Investor 1's optimal portfolio on the Markowitz efficient frontier will:
A. be the same as Investor 2's optimal portfolio.
B. have less risk than Investor 2's optimal portfolio.
C. have more risk than Investor 2's optimal portfolio.

81. Greg Burns, CFA, manages a portfolio, P, with expected return equal to 10% and standard deviation equal to 20%. The risk-free rate is 5%. Burns advises Victoria Hull to invest 40% in portfolio P and the remainder in the risk-free asset. The standard deviation for Hull's overall investment will be:
A. 7%.
B. 8%.
C. 12%.

82. Endowments and foundations typically have investment needs that are *best* described as:
A. long time horizon, high risk tolerance, and low liquidity needs.
B. long time horizon, low risk tolerance, and high liquidity needs.
C. short time horizon, low risk tolerance, and low liquidity needs.

83. When performing strategic asset allocation, properly defined and specified asset classes should:
A. have high returns correlations with other asset classes.
B. approximate the investor's total investable universe as a group.
C. each contain assets that have a broad range of risk and expected return.

84. The standard deviation of returns for a portfolio of risky assets is:
A. less than the standard deviation of the least risky asset.
B. greater than the standard deviation of the least risky asset.
C. less than or equal to the standard deviation of the most risky asset.

Questions 85 through 96 relate to Equity Investments. (18 minutes)

85. One of the functions of secondary markets is that they:
A. provide liquidity, and a financial futures contract is an example of a security trading on such a market.
B. provide liquidity, and a private placement is an example of a security trading on such a market.
C. provide fees, and a financial futures contract is an example of a security trading on such a market.

86. Mike Bowers observes that during one year the return on the S&P 500 index is 20%. Recalculating the return on an equally weighted basis, Bowers estimates that the index return is 15%. The difference in the two calculations of return is *best* explained by:
A. large capitalization stocks outperforming small capitalization stocks.
B. small capitalization stocks outperforming large capitalization stocks.
C. dividends on the stocks in the index.

87. An analyst develops the following information to value a common stock.

- Last year's earnings per share = $4.00
- Real risk-free rate = 4%
- Inflation premium = 5%
- Return on equity (ROE), expected to remain constant in the future = 10%
- Dividend payout, expected to remain stable in the future = 30%
- Stock's beta = 1.4
- Expected market return = 14%

The value per share is *closest* to:
A. $14.39.
B. $21.28.
C. $31.39.

88. Ian Goode, CFA, is analyzing the price of the preferred stock of MegaGym. Goode estimates that MegaGym's earnings growth rate over the next five years will be 20%, and that MegaGym's earnings will then grow at a sustainable rate of 5%. The *most* appropriate method for Goode to value MegaGym's preferred stock is to:
A. use a historical price-to-earnings model.
B. use a multistage dividend discount model with 20% growth for five years and 5% thereafter.
C. divide the preferred dividend by the required rate of return on MegaGym's preferred stock.

89. A dark pool is *best* described as:
A. an exchange with low trading volume.
B. the loans underlying a mortgage-backed security.
C. an alternative trading system that does not reveal current orders.

90. Which of the following is *most likely* to increase a firm's return on equity?
A. Issuing new equity to retire debt.
B. Issuing new debt to retire common stock.
C. A decrease in the market value of its common stock.

91. Aros Funds manages a family of mutual funds and employs a team of fundamental analysts, who research firms by analyzing financial statements and SEC filings. Under which form(s) of the efficient market hypothesis (EMH) would Aros Funds have the potential to achieve positive risk-adjusted returns consistently using fundamental analysis?
    A. Weak form only.
    B. Semistrong form and weak form.
    C. No form of the EMH is consistent with earning positive risk-adjusted returns using fundamental analysis.

92. The national stock exchange in a developing country adopts regulations that prohibit insider trading. On balance, adopting these new regulations is *most likely* to:
    A. increase market efficiency.
    B. decrease market efficiency.
    C. have no significant effect on market efficiency.

93. As an analyst for Donavan Financial Advisors, Lou Marvin must estimate the appropriate inputs for the firm's equity valuation models. Donavan's preferred valuation model is the single-stage dividend discount model (DDM). Members of Marvin's valuation team have supplied him with several pieces of data related to Regional Utilities, including the company's earnings and dividends from the most recent year, the expected real risk-free rate, and the expected nominal growth in net income. To estimate the value of Regional Utilities, additional inputs to the DDM that will be necessary include the:
    A. price-to-cash flow ratio and the expected cash flow per share.
    B. expected rate of inflation and the expected earnings retention rate.
    C. historical growth rates in dividends and the required return on the Utility bond index.

94. An investor in a sponsored depository receipt (DR):
    A. holds the voting rights for the DR shares.
    B. must obtain the foreign currency in which the DR is traded.
    C. should be familiar with market procedures and regulations in the DR issuer's country.

95. Denver Savin, CFA, is an analyst for an investment boutique. Savin is considering investing in one of two companies, Delmar or Bell United. Savin's evaluation is based on his estimation of price to cash flow.

In millions, except for per-share items	*Delmar*	*Bell United*
Revenues	$3,000	$17,000
Taxes	$45	$600
Net income	$100	$1,500
Depreciation	$250	$800
Outstanding shares	100	500
Stock price per share	$25	$35

Based on the price to cash flow multiple, which stock is more attractive for purchase?
A. Delmar is more attractive.
B. Bell United is more attractive.
C. Delmar and Bell United are equally attractive.

96. James Martindale, CFA, manages a small mutual fund specializing in defensive stocks. For this fund, Martindale will buy stocks with:
A. high beta.
B. low systematic risk.
C. low price-to-earnings ratios.

Questions 97 through 110 relate to Fixed Income. (21 minutes)

97. Martina Profis runs a fixed-income portfolio for the pension fund of Whetherby Whittaker, Ltd. The portfolio contains a $12 million position in the corporate bonds of Dewey Treadmills. Profis is concerned that interest rates are likely to rise and has calculated that a 50 basis point increase in rates would cause a 4% decline in the Dewey bonds. The dollar duration of the position in Dewey Treadmills is *closest* to:
A. $96,000.
B. $480,000.
C. $960,000.

98. A 10-year, 5% bond is issued at a price to yield 5.2%. Three months after issuance, the yield on this bond has decreased by 100 basis points. The price of this bond at issuance and three months later is:
A. above par at issuance, but below par three months later.
B. below par at issuance, but above par three months later.
C. below par at issuance, and below par three months later.

99. An investment advisor states, "The return from investing in a bond consists of three parts: the coupon interest, the return of principal, and the capital gain or loss that the investor realizes on the bond." The advisor is:
A. correct.
B. incorrect, because these are not the only sources of return from investing in a bond.
C. incorrect, because an investor who holds a bond to maturity will not realize a capital gain or loss.

100. Based on the following rates:

1-year spot rate	2.0%
2-year spot rate	2.5%
3-year spot rate	3.0%
4-year spot rate	3.5%

The 2-year forward rate two years from now is *closest* to:
A. 3.25%.
B. 3.50%.
C. 4.50%.

101. Wendy Jones, CFA, is reviewing a current bond holding. The bond's duration is 10 and its convexity is 200. Jones believes that interest rates will decrease by 100 basis points. If Jones's forecast is accurate, the bond's price will change by approximately:
A. –8.0%.
B. +8.0%.
C. +12.0%.

102. Pat Murray, CFA, creates an index of 40 corporate bonds rated Aa2 and an index of 40 municipal bonds rated Aa2. Compared to bonds in the corporate bond index, the default rate for bonds in the municipal bond index is *most likely* to be:
A. lower.
B. higher.
C. the same.

103. Bartel Corp. is building a new manufacturing facility in a foreign country where production costs will be considerably less than costs at Bartel's aging domestic plant. Bartel expects the increased profits from this facility to return the cost of construction within seven years. Bartel hopes to finance the new facility with a single debt issue with the lowest cost. The form of borrowing *best* suited to meet this goal is:
A. medium-term notes.
B. debentures with a negative pledge clause.
C. secured mortgage bonds.

104. Jane Higgins, CFA, is analyzing a corporate bond that she believes is a suitable addition for a client's portfolio. The 10-year security has a 7.5% annual coupon and is non-callable. The bond is currently priced at 104.50 to yield 7.177%. According to Higgins's analysis, for a 25 basis point decrease in yield, the bond's price will increase to 107.42 and for a 25 basis point increase in yield, the bond's price will decrease to 101.38. Higgins's estimation of the bond's effective duration is *closest* to:
A. 5.8.
B. 10.0.
C. 11.6.

105. An annual-pay 5% coupon corporate bond with two years to maturity has a nominal spread to Treasuries of 125 basis points and a zero-volatility spread of 150 basis points. The 1-year Treasury spot rate is 3.5%, and the 2-year Treasury spot rate is 4.0%. The price of the corporate bond (as a percent of par) is *closest* to:
A. 99.10.
B. 99.55.
C. 101.90.

106. For three otherwise identical bonds, which feature would result in the largest increase in value during a period of rising interest rate volatility?
A. Put feature.
B. Call feature.
C. Floating rate coupon.

107. Gerald Snow is a bond manager for Long Vision Investments. Snow is evaluating potential arbitrage opportunities. He has the following list of bonds:
- Bond X is a 1-year zero coupon bond selling at 950.
- Bond Y is a 2-year zero coupon bond selling at 850.
- Bond Z is a 2-year bond with an annual coupon of 8%.

All three bonds have a par value of $1,000. If no arbitrage opportunity exists, the price of Bond Z is *closest* to:
A. $975.
B. $995.
C. $1,015.

108. Three bonds are available for purchase that are identical in all respects except the following:
- Bond X: Noncallable, accelerated sinking fund.
- Bond Y: Callable, accelerated sinking fund.
- Bond Z: Noncallable, no sinking fund.

The correct order for these three bonds, from highest yield to lowest yield, is:
A. Bond X; Bond Z; Bond Y.
B. Bond Y; Bond Z; Bond X.
C. Bond Y; Bond X; Bond Z.

109. The difference between on-the-run and off-the-run U.S. Treasury securities is that on-the-run Treasury securities are:
A. traded only in the primary market, while off-the-run Treasury securities are traded only in the secondary market.
B. generally less actively traded than off-the-run Treasury securities and provide less reliable market yields.
C. the most recently auctioned Treasury securities in each maturity, while off-the-run Treasury securities are issues auctioned previously.

110. The 8% McClintock bonds maturing in 10 years are currently trading at 97.55. These bonds are option-free and pay coupons semiannually. The McClintock bonds have a:
A. yield to maturity greater than 8.0%.
B. current yield less than 8.0%.
C. nominal yield greater than 8.2%.

Questions 111 through 116 relate to Derivatives. (9 minutes)

111. JonesCorp enters into a plain vanilla interest rate swap as the fixed-rate receiver. The swap has a tenor of four years and makes payments quarterly on a netted basis. At initiation, the LIBOR term structure is flat and LIBOR is equal to the swap fixed rate. JonesCorp will make a future net payment to the swap counterparty if the LIBOR term structure:
A. becomes upward sloping.
B. remains flat but shifts down.
C. becomes downward sloping.

112. Gretchen Miller has been analyzing options on the common stock of Spirit Electronics Group, which last traded for $25.96. Miller has collected the following data on put options for Spirit stock that expire in three months:

Strike	*Put Price*
22.50	0.25
25.00	0.65
27.50	2.00

Miller has been asked by her supervisor to determine the profit on a protective put strategy using a strike price of $25.00 if the stock price is $27.13 on the option expiration date. What figure should Miller report to her supervisor?
A. $0.00.
B. $0.52.
C. $0.65.

113. Black Oil is an oil and gas exploration and production company. Black's management hedges its crude oil production using futures contracts. To close out the futures position, Black is *least likely* to:
A. hold the cash settled future until expiration.
B. physically settle according to exchange rules.
C. offset the transaction by shorting the oil futures contract on the same exchange.

114. For a European-style put option with a strike price of $30 on a stock that is trading at $28, the theoretical minimum value prior to expiration is:
A. equal to the theoretical minimum value of an otherwise identical American put.
B. less than the theoretical minimum value of an otherwise identical American put.
C. greater than the theoretical minimum value of an otherwise identical American put.

115. An analyst is considering buying a call option on ZXC stock, which is currently trading at $33.75 per share. If three-month call options with a strike price of $30 are trading at a premium of $4.50:
A. the ZXC call options are currently out of the money.
B. the breakeven underlying price for ZXC stock is $38.25 per share.
C. the potential upside of the ZXC call options is unlimited.

116. Two junior portfolio managers at ContraFunds, a hedge fund manager, have been asked to summarize the mechanics of utilizing futures contracts for the firm's training manual. The first manager, Tina Kent, submits a paragraph explaining that administering a futures position will require bringing the margin account balance back to the initial margin level by posting maintenance margin any time the balance falls below the variation margin level. The second manager, Martin Ramsey, submits a paragraph explaining margin requirements are determined according to the daily settlement price, which is the average of the last few trades of the day. Are Kent and Ramsey correct with regard to their explanation of the mechanics of futures positions?
    A. Both of these managers are correct.
    B. Neither of these managers is correct.
    C. Only one of these managers is correct.

Questions 117 through 120 relate to Alternative Investments. (6 minutes)

117. The gold futures market is said to be in contango if prices for gold futures are currently:
    A. equal to the spot price.
    B. less than the spot price.
    C. greater than the spot price.

118. An investment in a hedge fund with a 2-and-20 fee structure has increased in value each period and earned a return of 8% net of management fees in 20x7. Under which of the following provisions would incentive fees for 20x7 be the highest?
    A. 5% hard hurdle rate and a high water mark provision.
    B. 6% soft hurdle rate and a high water mark provision.
    C. 7% hard hurdle rate and no high water mark provision.

119. An analyst using the comparable sales approach to value a real estate property should:
    A. consider the most recent sale price of the property.
    B. determine an appropriate discount rate for future cash flows from the property.
    C. adjust for differences between this property and others that have been sold recently.

120. A leveraged buyout fund is evaluating Siena Company relative to its peer companies. Siena is *most likely* a good candidate for a management buy-in if it has:
    A. higher cash flow and less capable managers than its peers.
    B. lower cash flow and more capable managers than its peers.
    C. higher cash flow and more capable managers than its peers.

End of Morning Session

Exam 1
Afternoon Session

Topic	Questions	Points
Ethical and Professional Standards	1–18	27
Quantitative Methods	19–32	21
Economics	33–44	18
Financial Reporting and Analysis	45–68	36
Corporate Finance	69–78	15
Portfolio Management	79–84	9
Equity Investments	85–96	18
Fixed Income	97–110	21
Derivatives	111–116	9
Alternative Investments	117–120	6
Total		**180**

Test Answers

1.	A	B	C	41.	A	B	C	81.	A	B	C
2.	A	B	C	42.	A	B	C	82.	A	B	C
3.	A	B	C	43.	A	B	C	83.	A	B	C
4.	A	B	C	44.	A	B	C	84.	A	B	C
5.	A	B	C	45.	A	B	C	85.	A	B	C
6.	A	B	C	46.	A	B	C	86.	A	B	C
7.	A	B	C	47.	A	B	C	87.	A	B	C
8.	A	B	C	48.	A	B	C	88.	A	B	C
9.	A	B	C	49.	A	B	C	89.	A	B	C
10.	A	B	C	50.	A	B	C	90.	A	B	C
11.	A	B	C	51.	A	B	C	91.	A	B	C
12.	A	B	C	52.	A	B	C	92.	A	B	C
13.	A	B	C	53.	A	B	C	93.	A	B	C
14.	A	B	C	54.	A	B	C	94.	A	B	C
15.	A	B	C	55.	A	B	C	95.	A	B	C
16.	A	B	C	56.	A	B	C	96.	A	B	C
17.	A	B	C	57.	A	B	C	97.	A	B	C
18.	A	B	C	58.	A	B	C	98.	A	B	C
19.	A	B	C	59.	A	B	C	99.	A	B	C
20.	A	B	C	60.	A	B	C	100.	A	B	C
21.	A	B	C	61.	A	B	C	101.	A	B	C
22.	A	B	C	62.	A	B	C	102.	A	B	C
23.	A	B	C	63.	A	B	C	103.	A	B	C
24.	A	B	C	64.	A	B	C	104.	A	B	C
25.	A	B	C	65.	A	B	C	105.	A	B	C
26.	A	B	C	66.	A	B	C	106.	A	B	C
27.	A	B	C	67.	A	B	C	107.	A	B	C
28.	A	B	C	68.	A	B	C	108.	A	B	C
29.	A	B	C	69.	A	B	C	109.	A	B	C
30.	A	B	C	70.	A	B	C	110.	A	B	C
31.	A	B	C	71.	A	B	C	111.	A	B	C
32.	A	B	C	72.	A	B	C	112.	A	B	C
33.	A	B	C	73.	A	B	C	113.	A	B	C
34.	A	B	C	74.	A	B	C	114.	A	B	C
35.	A	B	C	75.	A	B	C	115.	A	B	C
36.	A	B	C	76.	A	B	C	116.	A	B	C
37.	A	B	C	77.	A	B	C	117.	A	B	C
38.	A	B	C	78.	A	B	C	118.	A	B	C
39.	A	B	C	79.	A	B	C	119.	A	B	C
40.	A	B	C	80.	A	B	C	120.	A	B	C

Exam 1
Afternoon Session

Questions 1 through 18 relate to Ethical and Professional Standards. (27 minutes)

1. Tom Laird, CFA, subscribes to several different analytical and research reporting services, reviews their research, and presents the analysis he believes is accurate to his clients. Laird attributes the material to its sources. Laird's method of providing analysis to his clients:
   A. does not violate any Standards.
   B. violates the Standard on diligence and reasonable basis.
   C. violates the Standard related to independence and objectivity.

2. A GIPS-compliant composite must comprise:
   A. the best performing fee-paying discretionary portfolios.
   B. all discretionary portfolios managed with the same objective or strategy.
   C. all fee-paying discretionary portfolios managed with the same objective or strategy.

3. Isaac Jones, CFA, wishes to buy Maxima common stock for some of his clients' accounts. Jones also wishes to purchase Maxima for his personal account. In accordance with CFA Institute Standards, Jones:
   A. must disclose his personal account purchase, in writing and in advance, to his clients and employer.
   B. may purchase Maxima for his personal account, but the transactions for his clients must take priority.
   C. may purchase Maxima at any time, as long as the execution price is not more favorable than the execution price given to the clients.

4. Wallace Manaugh, CFA, is analyzing the stock of a manufacturer of fishing boats. By analyzing public information, speaking with the firm's suppliers and customers, and counting the new boats in the company's boat yard, Manaugh concludes that the company's new fishing boat is not meeting sales expectations. Anticipating that this will cause the stock price to decline, Manaugh takes a short position in the stock. Manaugh has:
   A. not violated CFA Institute Standards.
   B. violated the Standards by acting on nonpublic information.
   C. an obligation under the Standards to make reasonable efforts to achieve public dissemination of the nonpublic information.

5. Rob Tegger, CFA, manages the investment account of The Knox Trust. The trustees tell Tegger they are pleased the account has outperformed its benchmark for the first three quarters of the year and that if he can outperform the benchmark over the final quarter, the trust will pay all the expenses for a week's vacation for Tegger and his wife at a trust property on Maui. To comply with the Code and Standards, Tegger must:
   A. obtain permission from his employer before accepting the offer.
   B. reject the offer because it creates a conflict of interest with his other clients.
   C. inform his employer of the offer, but he is not required to obtain permission before accepting it.

6. According to the Standard concerning fair dealing, new or changed investment recommendations should be made available to:
   A. all clients.
   B. clients who have indicated a prior interest in that type of security.
   C. only clients who have selected a level of service that includes such notification.

7. Ron Rice, CFA, is a broker who has received a large sell order for shares of a small-cap stock from a mutual fund that is a large holder of the stock. Rice believes this will have a negative effect on the stock price because the mutual fund is widely respected and investors will view it as an indication that the fund has lost confidence in the stock. Rice adds his own 1,000 shares to the sell order of the fund when he sells the block. Rice has:
   A. violated the Standard regarding material nonpublic information.
   B. not violated the Standards since he added so few shares to the much larger order.
   C. violated the Standard regarding duties to clients, but not the Standard regarding nonpublic information.

8. In presenting the firm's investment results in compliance with GIPS, how should any firm-specific information be handled?
   A. When appropriate, it is acceptable to include any additional firm-specific information within the GIPS presentation.
   B. If there is firm-specific information that lies outside of GIPS, this information should be included in a report separate from the GIPS presentation of results.
   C. Because GIPS are intended to be a comprehensive set of guidelines, firm-specific information not required in the performance results should not be included.

9. Hugh Nelson, CFA, has recently been offered a supervisory role at his firm. Nelson will be responsible for managing a large staff of portfolio managers and securities analysts. Before accepting the position, Nelson reviews the firm's compliance policies and procedures. Nelson feels the procedures and policies are adequate, with one major exception, a trade allocation procedure. Nelson's *most* appropriate action is to:
   A. accept the position with the understanding that the trade allocation procedures will be fixed immediately.
   B. decline in writing to accept the promotion until adequate compliance procedures are in place.
   C. accept the position, implement an adequate trade allocation procedure, and encourage the firm to adopt policies consistent with CFA Institute Standards.

10. CFA Institute's Global Investment Performance Standards (GIPS) are performance presentation guidelines based on a standardized, industry-wide approach, and:
    A. are voluntary.
    B. the CFA Institute Code and Standards require the use of GIPS for both current and prospective clients.
    C. investment firms that follow the CFA Institute Code and Standards are required to use GIPS for existing, but not prospective, clients when presenting investment performance results.

11. Riley and Smith, a broker/dealer, is bringing to market a secondary offering for All Pro Company. One of the reasons All Pro selected the firm to lead the offering is because Riley and Smith has been a market maker for All Pro's stock for the past five years. The firm is in possession of material nonpublic information relevant to All Pro's offering. To be in compliance with the Code and Standards, Riley and Smith:
    A. may not serve as underwriter for the same stock in which it acts as a market maker.
    B. should continue to serve as market maker but take only the contra side of unsolicited customer trades.
    C. should abstain from making a market in All Pro stock during the offering period but may resume market making activities after the offering.

12. Andrew Pollard, CFA, manages several client accounts for Nasu Koin Investments. Pollard directs trades through a variety of brokerage firms. While he attempts to balance his use of brokerage firms, he tends to favor Timberlake Brokers. Although Timberlake is not the lowest price brokerage firm, Pollard finds the research they provide especially useful. In exchange for the business Timberlake is receiving from Nasu Koin, Timberlake recommends Pollard and Nasu Koin's investment services to some of its clients. According to the Standards of Professional Conduct, Pollard:
    A. does not need to take any further action to comply with the Standards.
    B. must disclose the referral arrangement with Timberlake to his employer and clients.
    C. has violated the Standard related to independence and objectivity by favoring Timberlake.

13. Which of the following statements is *least likely* to be consistent with the Standard on preservation of confidentiality?
    A. The confidentiality of client information is protected only for current clients of the member or candidate.
    B. When permissible under applicable law, a member or candidate may forward confidential information to the CFA Institute's Professional Conduct Program.
    C. If confidential information concerns illegal activities on the part of the client, the member or candidate may disclose such information to authorities unless applicable law prohibits such disclosure.

14. Versoxy Pharmaceuticals recently hired Meelono Investment Partners to work on a secondary public stock offering. Meelono's brokerage division currently has a "Hold" recommendation on Versoxy's stock. Ed Hall, investment banking head, asks Ward Lear, CFA, the head of the brokerage division, to change the recommendation to "Buy." Lear's *most* appropriate action is to:
    A. place Versoxy on a restricted list and give out only factual information about the firm.
    B. assign a different analyst to analyze Versoxy but not mention his conversation with Hall.
    C. direct the currently assigned analyst to re-examine Versoxy and consider changing the recommendation to "Buy."

15. Which of the following statements is *most* accurate regarding the GIPS requirement for definition of the firm?
    A. The firm must be the distinct business entity held out to clients.
    B. If a firm has offices in different geographical locations, the firm definition may include just the primary location where all the investment decisions are made.
    C. The firm definition may include the corporation or a subsidiary of the corporation, but the firm cannot be defined as simply a "division" of the corporation.

16. Janet Todd passed Level II of the CFA program in June of last year and wants to note on her résumé her involvement in the CFA program. Todd passed both Level I and Level II of the CFA examination on her first attempts and plans to register for the Level III examination next year. Which of the following is an acceptable reference to her participation in the CFA Program? Janet Todd:
    A. is a Level III Candidate in the CFA program.
    B. is a Level II CFA.
    C. passed the Level I and Level II CFA examinations on her first attempts.

17. Joe Anderson, after working for U.S. Securities for 20 years as an economist, leaves the firm. U.S. Securities wishes to retain Anderson's services as an independent contractor. Anderson agrees to provide U.S. Securities with research and will be compensated for each report. Anderson will work from home, using his own personal computer. Six months after the start of the arrangement, one of U.S. Securities' competitors contacts Anderson about providing similar analytical work for them. According to CFA Institute Standards of Professional Conduct, Anderson:
    A. may accept this additional work as long as he abides by the terms of his oral agreement with U.S. Securities.
    B. must disclose this potential conflict to U.S. Securities.
    C. must obtain consent from U.S. Securities before accepting the additional work.

18. Jerry Brock, CFA, is a partner in a small investment advisory firm that caters to high net worth individuals. He has experienced a number of personal and financial setbacks over the past two years and has filed for bankruptcy protection. Has Brock violated CFA Institute Standards of Professional Conduct?
    A. No, unless his personal financial difficulties result from actions that reflect adversely on his honestly and integrity.
    B. No, but he must disclose the bankruptcy filing to his clients.
    C. Yes, because a member must conduct both their personal and professional business in a manner that protects their reputation and integrity.

Questions 19 through 32 relate to Quantitative Methods. (21 minutes)

19. Zach Mann is examining stock performance after classifying stocks according to their market capitalization (firm size) and P/E ratio. First, Mann ranks stocks based on market capitalization by grouping stocks into deciles. Then, for each firm size decile, he classifies stocks into P/E ratio quintiles. The total number of classifications created by Mann equals:
    A. 5.
    B. 10.
    C. 50.

20. A continuous uniform distribution is bounded by zero and 20. The probability of an outcome equal to 12 is *closest* to:
    A. 0.00.
    B. 0.05.
    C. 0.60.

21. The chi-square test *least likely*:
    A. uses a distribution with a lower bound of zero.
    B. is used to test whether a variance equals a certain value.
    C. can be used to make inferences even if the population is not normally distributed.

22. Jeffrey Hogan is an analyst for Maine Investments. Hogan is convinced that technical analysts can provide superior investment advice to their clients. Hogan believes:
    - Technical analysis is not based on analysis of financial statements and thus is not bound by accounting conventions that can distort valuation results.
    - By focusing on investment sentiment factors, technical analysis can consider even irrational investor behavior.

    A technical analyst would *most likely* agree with:
    A. both of these statements.
    B. neither of these statements.
    C. only one of these statements.

23. An investor plans to divide her funds evenly between two assets. Assets 1 and 2 have standard deviations of 10% and 30%, respectively. If the two assets are perfectly positively correlated, the standard deviation of returns of the portfolio is *closest* to:
    A. 10%.
    B. 15%.
    C. 20%.

24. David McWyllie obtains the price-to-equity ratios and the debt-to-equity ratios for each of 1,000 U.K. companies, for a total of 1,000 paired observations for the same time period. Which of the following *best* characterizes the data examined by McWyllie?
A. Time-series.
B. Cross-sectional.
C. Stratified.

25. Dillon Marshall has determined that the weighted average cost of capital for WestStar, Inc., is 12%. WestStar is evaluating three capital investment projects with conventional cash flows. If Project 1 has a positive net present value (NPV), Project 2 has an NPV of zero, and Project 3 has a negative NPV:
A. Project 1 has an internal rate of return greater than the WACC.
B. Project 2 will increase the size and value of WestStar.
C. Project 3 assumes reinvestment at a rate higher than the WACC.

26. Jackson Aerospace offers a defined benefit pension to its retirees. To maintain its fully funded status, Jackson determines that the pension portfolio must earn at least 7% per year. The expected return and standard deviation for Jackson's pension portfolio returns are 15% and 4%, respectively. Assuming the portfolio returns are normally distributed, the pension fund's shortfall risk is *closest* to:
A. 2.5%.
B. 5.0%.
C. 15.0%.

27. An investment analyst is reviewing the performance of various asset classes. The table below details the performance of the asset classes for the past year.

Asset Class	*Real Estate*	*Fixed Income*	*Equities*
Mean return	25%	8%	20%
Standard deviation	18%	4%	15%

The risk-free rate is 4%. For these asset classes, the:
A. coefficient of variation for real estate is greater than that for equities.
B. Sharpe ratio for equities is less than that for fixed income.
C. coefficient of variation for fixed income is the lowest of all these asset classes.

28. Chester Murphy, CFA, is a stock analyst who screens stocks based on market capitalization and earnings momentum. Murphy selects stocks that have market capitalization less than $1 billion ("small cap") and that have 5-year annualized earnings growth of at least 25% ("high earnings momentum"). The probability that a randomly selected stock is a small cap stock is 20%. The probability that a company has high earnings momentum, given that it is a small cap stock, is 40%. The probability that a randomly selected stock meets both of Murphy's investment criteria is *closest* to:
A. 8%.
B. 12%.
C. 20%.

29. Brandon Ratliff, CFA, is investigating whether the mean of abnormal returns earned by portfolio managers with an MBA degree significantly differs from mean abnormal returns earned by managers without an MBA. Ratliff's null hypothesis is that the means are equal. If Ratliff's critical *t*-value is 1.98 and his computed *t*-statistic is 2.05, he should:
A. reject the null hypothesis and conclude that the population means are equal.
B. fail to reject the null hypothesis and conclude that the population means are equal.
C. reject the null hypothesis and conclude that the population means are not equal.

30. Lou Gold, CFA, is screening all stocks on an exchange and grouping them by the industry in which they operate. Gold then selects stocks at random from each industry and combines the selected stocks to form an index to represent the performance of all stocks on the exchange. Gold's screening process is *best* described as:
A. simple random sampling.
B. systematic random sampling.
C. stratified sampling.

31. An analyst for Byg Investments, Inc., is attempting to visually demonstrate the dispersion of quarterly GDP growth for the last 60 years. The analyst should *most* appropriately employ a:
A. variance polygon.
B. histogram.
C. time series plot.

32. Cindy Jager, CFA, examines profits for 100 venture capital investments. The sample average profit is $2 million, and the sample standard deviation is $50 million. A 90% confidence interval for the population mean venture capital profit is *closest* to:
A. –$80.5 million to $84.5 million.
B. –$8 million to $12 million.
C. –$6.25 million to $10.25 million.

Questions 33 through 44 relate to Economics. (18 minutes)

33. Assume that the long-term equilibrium money market interest rate is 4% and the current money market interest rate is 3%. At this current rate of 3%, there will be an excess:
    A. demand for money in the money market, and investors will tend to be net buyers of securities.
    B. demand for money in the money market, and investors will tend to be net sellers of securities.
    C. supply of money in the money market, and investors will tend to be net buyers of securities.

34. A central bank that wants to increase short-term interest rates is *most likely* to:
    A. sell government securities.
    B. issue long-term bonds.
    C. decrease bank reserve requirements.

35. Under which of the following exchange rate regimes do the actions of a country's monetary authority keep the domestic currency closest to its stated target exchange rate with another currency?
    A. Fixed peg.
    B. Dollarization.
    C. Currency board.

36. A firm operating in an industry characterized by monopolistic competition will *least likely*:
    A. earn positive economic profits in the short run.
    B. maximize economic profits by colluding with the other firms and operating as a single seller.
    C. differentiate its product based on price or quality.

37. Jasmir Singh, CFA, is discussing unemployment and makes the following statements:
    - Frictional unemployment describes unemployment resulting from economic cycles. When the economy goes into a recession, frictional unemployment increases.
    - Structural unemployment results from a mismatch between workers' skills and the jobs available as economic changes eliminate some jobs and create new ones.

    Has Singh accurately described these two types of unemployment?
    A. Both of these statements are accurate.
    B. Neither of these statements is accurate.
    C. Only one of these statements is accurate.

38. Hanover Industrial operates a factory in Paris, which produces goods at a marginal cost above marginal revenue, and a factory in Munich, which products identical goods at a marginal cost less than marginal revenue. To maximize profits, Hanover should *most likely*:
   A. decrease output at both factories.
   B. decrease output at the Paris factory and increase output at the Munich factory.
   C. increase output at the Paris factory and decrease output at the Munich factory.

39. When two goods are complements, the cross elasticity of demand is:
   A. positive, and for substitutes the cross price elasticity of demand is negative.
   B. negative, and for substitutes the cross price elasticity of demand is negative.
   C. negative, and for substitutes the cross price elasticity of demand is positive.

40. Compared to a competitive market result, a single-price monopolist will *most likely*:
   A. adopt a marginal cost pricing strategy, which will decrease consumer surplus.
   B. increase price, decrease consumer surplus, and increase producer surplus.
   C. reduce output, create a deadweight loss, and decrease both producer and consumer surplus.

41. With regard to the balance of payments, the purchase of rights to natural resources in a country by foreigners would be *most likely* to affect the country's:
   A. capital account.
   B. current account.
   C. financial account.

42. At the quantities where the marginal cost curve intersects the average variable cost (AVC) curve and the average total cost (ATC) curve, respectively:
    A. AVC and ATC are at their minimum points.
    B. AVC is at its minimum point and ATC is increasing.
    C. ATC is at its minimum point and AVC is decreasing.

43. The ability to trade goods and services indirectly in an economy that uses money, as compared to trading them directly in an economy that uses barter, results from which of the three basic functions of money?
    A. Store of value.
    B. Unit of account.
    C. Medium of exchange.

44. Fiscal policy will result in the largest increase in aggregate demand if the government increases:
    A. taxes only.
    B. spending only.
    C. spending and taxes equally.

Questions 45 through 68 relate to Financial Reporting and Analysis. (36 minutes)

45. Information about the operating profits of a company's various business segments can be found in the:
    A. proxy statement.
    B. auditor's report.
    C. supplementary schedules.

46. The following financial information reflects the latest 12-month results for High Corp (in millions):

Revenue	$400
Expenses	$300
Liabilities	$350
Dividends paid	$10
Beginning retained earnings	$125
Ending retained earnings	$215
Contributed capital	$175

    High Corp's assets are *closest* to:
    A. $565 million.
    B. $650 million.
    C. $740 million.

47. Stone Development Company owns four office buildings and a tract of raw land. Stone occupies one of the buildings, collects rental income from the other three buildings, and is holding the land for capital appreciation. Under IFRS, which of these assets should Stone classify as investment property on its balance sheet?
A. All of these assets.
B. Only the land held for capital appreciation.
C. The land and the buildings that generate rental income.

48. Lyon Company had pretax earnings of $150 million in its first year of operation. Pretax income included:
- $25 million of interest income from tax-free municipal bonds.
- $35 million of accrued warranty expense that is not yet deductible.
- $15 million of deductible depreciation expense that is not yet accrued.

At a tax rate of 40%, Lyon's income taxes payable are:
A. $58 million.
B. $60 million.
C. $70 million.

49. For a firm that reports under IFRS, required disclosures related to inventories *most likely* include:
A. effects on income from liquidating inventory.
B. circumstances of any reversals of inventory writedowns.
C. the difference between inventory values under LIFO and FIFO.

50. The proper treatment for a change in accounting principle is to:
A. restate the current period's financial statements and disclose the effect of the change in the footnotes.
B. restate financial statements for all periods included in the company's financial statements.
C. include the cumulative effect of the changes on the financial statements and describe the effects of the new standard compared to the old one in the footnotes.

51. Bay Airlines leases a fleet of 100 airplanes used to transport freight. Bay structures the terms of all aircraft leases such that the leases are classified as operating leases. Annual lease payments for Bay's latest airplane acquisition is $1,000. If the company were to capitalize the lease, the reclassification would effectively increase interest expense by $600 and amortization expense by $450. Under U.S. GAAP, the effect of capitalizing the lease on Bay's cash flow is:
A. a reduction of cash flow from operations.
B. a reduction of cash flow from financing.
C. an increase in cash flow from investing.

52. A company fails to accrue wages for December that will be paid in January. The company's year-end balance sheet liabilities:
A. and assets are understated.
B. are overstated and owners' equity is understated.
C. are understated and owners' equity is overstated.

53. At the end of 20X8, Wichita, Inc., purchased equipment totaling $500,000. The seller of the equipment provided 100% debt financing with payments, including interest, that begin in 20X9. How does the equipment purchase affect Wichita's 20X8 cash flows?
A. No effect.
B. Decrease cash flow from operations.
C. Decrease cash flow from investment.

54. Which of the following analyst adjustments to improve comparability among firms' financial statements is *most accurate*?
A. Subtract goodwill from a firm's assets.
B. Add the change in the LIFO reserve to a firm's cost of goods sold.
C. Add the sum of the disclosed payment obligations on operating leases to a firm's liabilities.

55. The major benefit of reporting standards is that they:
A. prevent management from manipulating financial results.
B. ensure that financial reports are usable by a wide range of audiences.
C. enable direct comparisons between companies by requiring them to use standard formats and methods.

56. If a firm's management wants to use its discretion over accounting choices to increase operating income in the next period, they are *most likely* to:
A. decrease the assumed useful lives of plant and equipment.
B. increase the assumed residual values of plant and equipment.
C. write up plant and equipment from depreciated cost to its fair market value.

57. Peney, Inc., is building a new office tower for its administrative personnel. The construction costs are funded using a combination of debt and equity. As compared to expensing the construction costs immediately, capitalizing the construction costs will result in:
A. a higher interest coverage ratio and lower operating cash flow.
B. higher total assets and higher financing cash flow.
C. a lower fixed asset turnover ratio and lower investing cash flow.

58. Selected financial ratios for three firms in the same industry appear in the following table:

	Kovacs Co.	*Linwood Co.*	*McDowell Co.*
Debt-to-equity	0.3×	0.6×	0.6×
Interest coverage	3.5×	5.0×	3.5×
Fixed charge coverage	1.6×	1.6×	3.2×

Based only on these ratios, the *most* solvent of these firms is:
A. Kovacs.
B. Linwood.
C. McDowell.

59. To compute cash collections from customers when converting a statement of cash flows from the indirect to the direct method, an analyst begins with:
A. net income and adds back non-cash expenses.
B. sales, subtracts any increase in accounts receivable, and adds any increase in unearned revenue.
C. cost of goods sold, subtracts any increase in accounts payable, adds any increase in inventory, and subtracts any inventory write-offs.

60. Magnus Aerospace produces and sells aircraft and has approximately a 2-year operating cycle. Magnus's liabilities include commercial paper due in 270 days, a bank note due in one year, and bonds that will mature in 18 months. Magnus should *most* appropriately classify as current liabilities:
A. all of these liabilities.
B. only the commercial paper.
C. the commercial paper and the bank note.

61. Manitou Plastics, Inc., has been recording large deferred tax assets after incurring operating losses in the previous three years. At the end of the most recent year, Manitou reported $14 million in deferred tax assets but only $3 million in deferred tax liabilities. Manitou has also reported a valuation allowance related to deferred taxes in the amount of $7.5 million. What is the *most likely* cause of Manitou's reported valuation allowance?
A. Accounting earnings have been manipulated.
B. Future profitability is in doubt.
C. Interest rates have increased.

62. Barnes Company issues bonds to fund a capital spending program. The $200 million offering has a coupon rate of 6.0% and the bonds yield 6.5% at issuance. If the bonds' yield declines to 5.5% at the end of the year, reported interest expense will be:
A. less than $12 million.
B. more than $12 million.
C. exactly $12 million.

63. An analyst is responsible for evaluating the inventory accounting of companies in the finished lumber industry. The analyst is interested in two companies, Harrelson Lumber and Wilson Company. Harrelson and Wilson are identical in all respects except that Harrelson uses FIFO and Wilson uses LIFO. Inventory information for both companies is presented below:

	Units	Cost per unit
Beginning inventory	100	$10
First purchase	20	$8
Second purchase	30	$12
Third purchase	10	$6
Ending inventory	50	

Which of the following statements is *most* accurate?
A. Harrelson's cost of goods sold is lower than Wilson's.
B. Wilson's ending inventory is higher than Harrelson's.
C. Harrelson's and Wilson's cost of goods sold are the same.

64. McLoone Company's basic earnings per share are £1.20. McLoone has £10 million par value of 5% preference shares outstanding that can be converted into 400,000 common shares. Is McLoone required to report diluted earnings per share?
A. Yes, because the preference shares are dilutive to EPS.
B. No, because the preference shares are not dilutive to EPS.
C. Yes, because the preference shares are potentially dilutive to EPS.

65. Regarding the use of financial ratios in the analysis of a firm's financial statements, it is *most* accurate to say that:
A. many financial ratios are useful in isolation.
B. variations in accounting treatments have little effect on financial ratios.
C. a range of target values for a ratio may be more appropriate than a single target value.

66. Items that appear in other comprehensive income, but are excluded from the income statement, include:
A. losses due to expropriation of assets.
B. gains and losses due to foreign currency translation.
C. unrealized gains and losses on available-for-trading securities.

67. How is the impact of selling a long-lived asset recorded on a firm's income statement?
    A. The sale proceeds increase revenue and the carrying value increases cost of goods sold.
    B. The difference between the sale proceeds and the carrying value is reported as a gain or loss.
    C. The difference between the sale proceeds and the original value is reported as a gain or loss.

68. A company reports its financial statements according to International Financial Reporting Standards. The company's cash flow statement will report interest paid in either the:
    A. operating or investing section.
    B. investing or financing section.
    C. operating or financing section.

Questions 69 through 78 relate to Corporate Finance. (15 minutes)

69. The Garden and Home Store recently issued preferred stock paying \$2 annual dividends. The price of its preferred stock is \$20. The after-tax cost of fixed-rate debt capital is 6% and the cost of common stock equity is 12%. The cost of preferred stock is *closest* to:
    A. 9%.
    B. 10%.
    C. 11%.

70. William Mason, CFA, is a project manager for the semiconductor division of Mammoth Industries, a conglomerate. The semiconductor division's projected cash flows are less certain than Mammoth's overall cash flows. When determining the net present values of projects within the semiconductor division, Mason should use:
    A. Mammoth Industries' marginal cost of capital.
    B. a lower marginal cost of capital than Mammoth Industries.
    C. a higher marginal cost of capital than Mammoth Industries.

71. Bear Company produces gravel-hauling equipment. The company recently began producing the Mauler, a new line of equipment. Prior to beginning production of the Mauler, the company spent \$10 million in research and development costs. Bear expects the Mauler line to generate positive cash flows beginning in the fourth year. However, Bear is forecasting a one-time expense in year 5 to comply with new government emission standards. The company will use an empty building it already owns to produce the Mauler. When analyzing the project cash flows for the Mauler, Bear should *least* appropriately include the:
    A. research and development cost.
    B. compliance cost for emissions standards.
    C. use of the empty building.

72. A company is evaluating the following capital projects for investment over the next two years:
    - Two new machines with costs of $4 million each.
    - Computer software upgrade with a cost of $1 million.
    - Multi-year replacement of two aging machines involving an investment of $4.5 million for the first machine and another $4.5 million for the second machine if projected savings from the first machine are realized.

    All of these projects have positive net present values and the available budget is $10 million. The company should accept:
    A. all of these projects.
    B. those projects with the highest expected rates of return over the 2-year capital budgeting period.
    C. those projects with the highest present value of expected future cash flows relative to required investment.

73. A graph that shows the relation between the cost of capital and the value that a project adds to the firm is *best* described as a project's:
    A. characteristic line.
    B. net present value profile.
    C. marginal cost of capital curve.

74. Which of the following working capital management outcomes is *least* desirable?
    A. Low operating cycle.
    B. High inventory turnover.
    C. High cash conversion cycle.

75. A company's schedule of the costs of debt and equity shows that an additional $3 million of debt can be issued at an after-tax cost of 3%, and additional equity of $9 million can be issued at a cost of 6%. The company plans to maintain a capital structure of 30% debt and 70% equity. At what level of new capital financing will the marginal cost of capital change with the issuance of new debt?
    A. $3 million.
    B. $10 million.
    C. $13 million.

76. Avery Williams is a member of the board of directors for a pharmaceutical company. Shareowners should *most likely* view Williams as possessing the experience required to serve on the board if he has:
    A. served as an executive of the firm.
    B. served on the board for more than ten years.
    C. significant experience in financial operations and accounting.

77. Inventory turnover rates for a company were 8.3x in year 1, 8.1x in year 2, and 7.6x in year 3. The number of days of inventory for the industry averaged 50 in year 1, 49 in year 2, and 48 in year 3. The company's inventory management has been:
A. in line with the industry average in each year.
B. improving over the last three years.
C. worsening over the last three years.

78. Elenore Rice, CFA, is asked to determine the appropriate weighted average cost of capital for Samson Brick Company. Rice is provided with the following data:

Debt outstanding, market value	\$10 million
Common stock outstanding, market value	\$30 million
Marginal tax rate	40%
Cost of common equity	12%
Cost of debt	8%

Samson has no preferred stock. Assuming Samson's ratios reflect the firm's target capital structure, Samson's weighted average cost of capital is *closest* to:
A. 9.8%.
B. 10.2%.
C. 10.4%.

Questions 79 through 84 relate to Portfolio Management. (9 minutes)

79. Which of the following pooled investments is likely to require the smallest minimum investment amount?
A. Wrap fee account.
B. Market neutral fund.
C. Closed-end mutual fund.

80. All portfolios that lie on the capital market line:
A. contain the same mix of risky assets unless only the risk-free asset is held.
B. have some unsystematic risk unless only the risk-free asset is held.
C. contain at least some positive allocation to the risk-free asset.

81. The problem of investment managers taking offsetting active positions is *most likely* addressed by employing:
A. risk budgeting.
B. tactical asset allocation.
C. a core-satellite approach.

82. Stephanie Dell is evaluating two stocks (X and Y) using the capital asset pricing model. Dell predicts that the betas for the two stocks will be identical but that the unsystematic risk for Stock X will be much higher than for Stock Y. According to the capital asset pricing model, in equilibrium:
    A. Stock X will have a higher expected return than Stock Y but a standard deviation equal to Stock Y.
    B. Stock X will have a higher standard deviation than Stock Y but an expected return equal to Stock Y.
    C. both the expected return and standard deviation for Stock X will be higher than Stock Y.

83. In the Markowitz framework, risk is defined as the:
    A. variance of returns.
    B. probability of a loss.
    C. beta of an investment.

84. The covariance of monthly returns for two stocks is 0.91. Based on the covariance, it is *most* accurate to conclude that the monthly returns on these two stocks have:
    A. no linear relationship.
    B. a strong linear relationship.
    C. a positive linear relationship.

Questions 85 through 96 relate to Equity Investments. (18 minutes)

85. Sam Grant, CFA, publishes the Grant 50 Index, which consists of value stocks with small market capitalizations. The Grant 50 Index is best described as a:
    A. style index.
    B. sector index.
    C. value weighted index.

86. An investor who takes a short position in a stock is *least likely* to:
    A. borrow the stock from another investor.
    B. reinvest any dividend payments.
    C. post margin with his brokerage firm.

87. A buy side analyst is discussing the relative functionality of a stock market with her colleagues. She says, "This should be considered a well-functioning stock market because it is characterized by (1) rapid adjustment of prices to reflect new information and (2) low transactions costs that have little impact on prices." Are these accurate descriptions of attributes of a well-functioning market?
    A. Both descriptions are accurate.
    B. Neither description is accurate.
    C. Only one of these descriptions is accurate.

88. In an informationally efficient capital market, a portfolio manager who follows an active investment strategy is *most likely* to:
A. outperform a passive index strategy on average over time.
B. underperform a passive index strategy on average over time.
C. earn the same net return over time as a passive index strategy.

89. An increase in a firm's return on equity above investors' required rate of return on the firm's common stock, if it is expected to persist, will:
A. not have a predictable effect on market or book value.
B. increase both the firm's market value and its book value.
C. increase investors' required rate of return on the company's shares.

90. Holding other factors constant, a stock's expected price-to-earnings ratio:
A. decreases as the difference between the required rate of return on the stock and the expected constant growth rate of dividends widens.
B. decreases as the expected constant growth rate of dividends increases.
C. increases as the expected dividend payout ratio decreases.

91. Jack George, CFA, is evaluating Dunger, Inc., a waste management firm. The company has been experiencing a strong 15% growth rate, which is forecast to continue over the next three years before growth slows to a sustainable rate of 8%. The company recently paid a dividend of $0.50 per share. George has calculated a 10% weighted average cost of capital for Dunger. The firm has no debt. The company's last reported trade was $35 per share. Based on the multi-stage dividend discount model, George should:
A. not buy the stock.
B. buy the stock because its intrinsic value is $38 per share.
C. buy the stock because its intrinsic value is $41 per share.

92. Which type of stock index must be adjusted for stock splits?
A. Equal weighted index.
B. Price weighted index.
C. Market capitalization weighted index.

93. Acquire Corp. has a business model based on making accretive acquisitions each year. The company has historically been successful in implementing its strategy. Earnings per share have grown each of the last five years at a 15% compounded rate. Acquire's two primary business segments are engineering construction and mining. During the past year, Acquire purchased a services company with large net operating losses. The purchase price was one-half the company's current market value. The *most appropriate* technique to value Acquire is based on its:
A. price-to-book value ratio.
B. forward price-to-earnings ratio.
C. trailing price-to-sales ratio.

94. Which of the following limit orders is *least likely* to be filled?
A. Inside-the-market limit sell order.
B. Behind-the-market limit buy order.
C. Aggressively priced limit buy order.

95. Firms' pricing power is likely to be strongest in an industry that is characterized by:
A. overcapacity and high concentration.
B. undercapacity and high barriers to entry.
C. low barriers to entry and low concentration.

96. Liquidity is generally supplied by dealers in a:
A. brokered market.
B. order-driven market.
C. quote-driven market.

Questions 97 through 110 relate to Fixed Income. (21 minutes)

97. A bond initially does not make periodic payments but instead accrues them over a pre-determined period and then pays a lump sum at the end of that period. The bond subsequently makes regular periodic payments until maturity. Such a bond is *best* described as a:
A. step-up note.
B. zero-coupon bond.
C. deferred-coupon bond.

98. George Worrell, CFA, is valuing a U.S. Treasury bond using several scenarios and is interested in the impact of yield volatility. If Worrell assumes yield volatility increases, and holds all else constant, the estimated value for the bond will:
A. increase.
B. decrease.
C. remain the same.

99. Phillip Green, CFA, expects a downward trend in interest rates to reverse next month. Green believes that, in 30 days, interest rates will begin to rise steadily and significantly for at least 12 months. Green is evaluating three bonds for potential investment:

Bond	*Duration*	*Convexity*	*Maturity*	*Coupon*
A	8.0	0.153	12 yrs	7.0%
B	4.5	0.235	5 yrs	6.0%
C	7.2	0.212	9 yrs	5.5%

Based on his expectations, if Green invests in only one of these bonds, he should choose:
A. Bond A.
B. Bond B.
C. Bond C.

100. A company desiring to issue a fixed-income security has placed $10 million worth of loan receivables in a special purpose vehicle (SPV) that is independent of the issuer. The credit rating agencies suggest the company secure a third-party guarantee in order to have the security rated AAA. After completing the transfer of assets to the SPV and obtaining a letter of credit from a national bank, the company issues the AAA rated security. The securities are *most likely*:
A. commercial paper.
B. international bonds.
C. asset-backed securities.

101. A fixed-income portfolio manager is considering adding a security to his existing portfolio. The bond has an option adjusted spread (OAS) equal to 0.23% and a *Z*-spread equal to 0.15%. The manager believes this bond is a sound investment but is concerned that his portfolio is dominated by callable bonds. Therefore, the manager will only buy the bond if it is not callable. Should the manager add the bond to his portfolio?
A. Yes, the negative option cost implies the bond is putable.
B. No, the positive option cost implies the bond is callable.
C. No, the negative option cost implies the bond is callable.

102. If inflation is expected to remain at zero, the pure expectations theory and the liquidity preference theory, respectively, predict that the yield curve will be:

	Pure expectations	Liquidity preference
A.	Flat	Flat
B.	Upward sloping	Flat
C.	Flat	Upward sloping

103. On Monday, the yield curve is upward sloping with yields of 3%, 4%, and 5.5% on 1-year, 5-year, and 10-year Treasuries, respectively. The following day, the Treasury yield curve experiences an upward parallel shift equal to 112 basis points. Other things equal, which of the following noncallable 6% coupon bonds is likely to experience the smallest percent change in price as a result of the yield curve shift?
A. Corporate bond maturing in ten years.
B. Corporate bond maturing in five years.
C. U.S. Treasury bond maturing in ten years.

104. A bond dealer determines that the present value of a particular Treasury note, based on Treasury spot rates, is greater than its market price. The dealer can generate an arbitrage profit (assuming no transactions costs) by:
A. buying the Treasury note and selling its cash flows as Treasury STRIPS.
B. buying the equivalent Treasury STRIPS and selling them as a Treasury note.
C. buying the undervalued note and selling short the Treasury security with the nearest maturity.

105. Ann Lloyd, CFA, observes that a 3-year senior unsecured bond of Hawk, Inc. has a rating of Baa3/BBB– and a 3-year senior unsecured bond of Osprey, Inc. has a rating of Ba1/BB+. Based only on this information, Lloyd can *most appropriately* conclude that:
A. Credit risk is greater for the Osprey bond than for the Hawk bond.
B. Loss severity is greater for the Osprey bond than for the Hawk bond.
C. The Hawk bond is investment grade and the Osprey bond is non-investment grade.

106. Based on the following rates:

1-year spot rate	3.0%
1-year forward rate one year from now	5.0%
2-year forward rate one year from now	6.5%

The 3-year spot rate is *closest* to:
A. 5.0%.
B. 5.3%.
C. 9.3%.

107. A bond has a nominal spread to Treasuries of 150 basis points, a zero volatility spread of 130 basis points, and an option-adjusted spread of 90 basis points. It is *most likely* that the:
A. bond is putable.
B. bond is callable.
C. option cost is 20 basis points.

108. Rob Ealey, CFA, purchases an option-free bond with a 6.5% coupon that is currently selling at 94.73 to yield 7.25%. If yields increase by 50 basis points, the new price of the bonds would be 91.41, and if yields decrease by 50 basis points, the new price of the bond would be 98.20. If yields decrease by 75 basis points, the price of the bond would be *closest* to:
A. 89.64.
B. 99.82.
C. 104.92.

109. Debbie Scott, CFA, is planning to purchase a bond that matures in ten years, pays a 7% semiannual coupon, and is currently priced to yield 6.25%. The bond is callable at par beginning five years from now. Scott can reinvest coupon income from the bond at 5.5%. Which of the following statements is *least accurate*?
A. If the bond is called in six years, Scott's return will be less than 6.25%.
B. If Scott's reinvestment rate was 6.25%, the bond's yield to worst would be less than 6.25%.
C. If the bond was priced to yield 5.5%, the current yield would be 7%.

110. Richard Wallace manages a portfolio of fixed-income securities for a large multinational investment firm. Wallace's portfolio is exposed to reinvestment risk, which he is attempting to reduce by adding securities with low levels of reinvestment risk. Of the following bonds, Wallace should *most* appropriately choose:
A. a mortgage-backed security with scheduled principal and interest payments.
B. an 8%, 10-year Treasury bond with semiannual payments.
C. a 15-year Treasury STRIP.

Questions 111 through 116 relate to Derivatives. (9 minutes)

111. Peter Ulrich, CFA, runs a hedge fund which specializes in using option strategies to enhance the fund's returns. In a training session for newly hired analysts, Ulrich explains option characteristics as follows:
- The maximum profit on a short call position can be greater than the maximum profit on a long call position.
- A long at-the-money put option position will break even as soon as the price of the underlying stock decreases.

Are Ulrich's statements accurate?
A. Both of these statements are accurate.
B. Neither of these statements is accurate.
C. Only one of these statements is accurate.

112. Jack Cheney, CFA, purchases a Swenson, Inc., October 80 put option for a premium of $5. Cheney holds the option until the expiration date when Swenson stock sells for $78 per share. At expiration, the loss on the contract is:
  A. $2.
  B. $3.
  C. $5.

113. An equity portfolio combined with long puts will have profit and loss characteristics similar to a:
  A. long call option.
  B. short put and long call.
  C. covered call position.

114. A trader writes a put option on Treasury bond futures. If the option is exercised, the writer has an obligation to:
  A. buy Treasury bonds.
  B. take a long position in Treasury bond futures.
  C. take a short position in Treasury bond futures.

115. A European call option on Hartco stock with an exercise price of $50 and an expiration date one year from now is worth $4.00 today. A European put option on Hartco stock with an exercise price of $50 and an expiration date one year from now is worth $2.25 today. The risk-free rate for one year is 2.0%. The value of Hartco's stock is *closest* to:
  A. $43 per share.
  B. $47 per share.
  C. $51 per share.

116. Pamela Burke is a cotton farmer. Her crop will be ready for harvest in three months, but Burke does not believe prices will remain at their current level. Burke contacts Brooke Anderson, a derivatives dealer, to negotiate a forward contract. Anderson agrees to be the counterpart to a forward contract that will eliminate Burke's exposure to the price of cotton. The contract is structured as a nondeliverable forward with a contract price of $47. If the price of cotton is $49 in three months, which counterparty will be exposed to the greater amount of credit risk and which counterparty will make a payment?
  A. Burke will be exposed to greater credit risk, and Anderson will make a payment.
  B. Anderson will be exposed to greater credit risk, and Burke will make a payment.
  C. Burke will make a payment, but neither party is exposed to credit risk.

Questions 117 through 120 relate to Alternative Investments. (6 minutes)

117. A hedge fund that uses a market neutral strategy is *most likely* to have approximately equal investments in:
A. long and short equities.
B. equities, fixed income, and cash.
C. domestic and international markets.

118. Measures of downside risk such as the Sortino ratio are *most likely* to be more appropriate than standard deviation for measuring risk of a:
A. macro strategy fund.
B. real estate investment trust.
C. commodity exchange-traded fund.

119. Arkex Funds is a hedge fund with a value of $100 million at the beginning of the year. Arkex Funds charges a 2.0% management fee based on assets under management at the beginning of the year and a 20.0% incentive fee with a 5.0% hard hurdle rate. Incentive fees are calculated net of management fees. The value of the fund at the end of the year before fees is $110 million. The net return to investors is *closest to*:
A. 6.8%.
B. 7.4%
C. 8.0%.

120. If the futures market for a commodity is in backwardation, roll yield will be:
A. zero.
B. positive.
C. negative.

End of Afternoon Session

Exam 2
Morning Session

Topic	Questions	Points
Ethical and Professional Standards	1–18	27
Quantitative Methods	19–32	21
Economics	33–44	18
Financial Reporting and Analysis	45–68	36
Corporate Finance	69–78	15
Portfolio Management	79–84	9
Equity Investments	85–96	18
Fixed Income	97–110	21
Derivatives	111–116	9
Alternative Investments	117–120	6
Total		**180**

Test Answers

1.	A	B	C
2.	A	B	C
3.	A	B	C
4.	A	B	C
5.	A	B	C
6.	A	B	C
7.	A	B	C
8.	A	B	C
9.	A	B	C
10.	A	B	C
11.	A	B	C
12.	A	B	C
13.	A	B	C
14.	A	B	C
15.	A	B	C
16.	A	B	C
17.	A	B	C
18.	A	B	C
19.	A	B	C
20.	A	B	C
21.	A	B	C
22.	A	B	C
23.	A	B	C
24.	A	B	C
25.	A	B	C
26.	A	B	C
27.	A	B	C
28.	A	B	C
29.	A	B	C
30.	A	B	C
31.	A	B	C
32.	A	B	C
33.	A	B	C
34.	A	B	C
35.	A	B	C
36.	A	B	C
37.	A	B	C
38.	A	B	C
39.	A	B	C
40.	A	B	C
41.	A	B	C
42.	A	B	C
43.	A	B	C
44.	A	B	C
45.	A	B	C
46.	A	B	C
47.	A	B	C
48.	A	B	C
49.	A	B	C
50.	A	B	C
51.	A	B	C
52.	A	B	C
53.	A	B	C
54.	A	B	C
55.	A	B	C
56.	A	B	C
57.	A	B	C
58.	A	B	C
59.	A	B	C
60.	A	B	C
61.	A	B	C
62.	A	B	C
63.	A	B	C
64.	A	B	C
65.	A	B	C
66.	A	B	C
67.	A	B	C
68.	A	B	C
69.	A	B	C
70.	A	B	C
71.	A	B	C
72.	A	B	C
73.	A	B	C
74.	A	B	C
75.	A	B	C
76.	A	B	C
77.	A	B	C
78.	A	B	C
79.	A	B	C
80.	A	B	C
81.	A	B	C
82.	A	B	C
83.	A	B	C
84.	A	B	C
85.	A	B	C
86.	A	B	C
87.	A	B	C
88.	A	B	C
89.	A	B	C
90.	A	B	C
91.	A	B	C
92.	A	B	C
93.	A	B	C
94.	A	B	C
95.	A	B	C
96.	A	B	C
97.	A	B	C
98.	A	B	C
99.	A	B	C
100.	A	B	C
101.	A	B	C
102.	A	B	C
103.	A	B	C
104.	A	B	C
105.	A	B	C
106.	A	B	C
107.	A	B	C
108.	A	B	C
109.	A	B	C
110.	A	B	C
111.	A	B	C
112.	A	B	C
113.	A	B	C
114.	A	B	C
115.	A	B	C
116.	A	B	C
117.	A	B	C
118.	A	B	C
119.	A	B	C
120.	A	B	C

Exam 2
Morning Session

Questions 1 through 18 relate to Ethical and Professional Standards. (27 minutes)

1. Moe Girard, CFA, works in a large group that decides on recommendations by consensus. Girard does not always agree with the group consensus, but he is confident in the group's analytical ability. To comply with the Code and Standards when the group issues a recommendation with which he disagrees, Girard:
   A. does not need to take any action.
   B. must request that his name be removed from the group's report.
   C. should include his independent opinion as an appendix to the group's report.

2. The primary principles on which the CFA Institute Bylaws and Rules of Procedure for Proceedings Related to Professional Conduct are based *least likely* include:
   A. fair process.
   B. confidentiality.
   C. global application.

3. David Martin, CFA, recently joined Arc Financial as a portfolio manager of an emerging markets mutual fund. For the past three years, he managed an emerging markets mutual fund for Landmark Investments. Upon Martin's arrival, Arc Financial announces to existing and prospective clients, "While at Landmark Investments, Martin was the senior portfolio manager of Alpha Emerging Markets Fund. In Martin's three years as manager, this fund outperformed its benchmark each year, as documented in recent reports by Landmark." Does this statement violate the CFA Institute Standard of Professional Conduct related to performance presentation?
   A. No.
   B. Yes, because the Standards prohibit showing past performance at a prior firm.
   C. Yes, because Arc must present at least five years of Martin's performance history.

4. The recommended procedures for the Standard on material nonpublic information state that a firm's internal information "firewall" should include:
   A. a prohibition against buying and selling when the firm possesses material nonpublic information.
   B. a reporting system in which authorized personnel review and approve interdepartmental communications.
   C. distribution of a restricted list to all employees in the relevant departments of the firm.

5. Isabella Wilson recently completed Level III of the CFA examination program and was awarded her CFA charter. Which of the following statements would comply with CFA Institute Standards?
   A. "Wilson is among the best analysts in her field, as shown by passing the three levels of the CFA exam in consecutive attempts."
   B. "Wilson recently passed Level III and received her CFA, having passed all three levels in consecutive attempts."
   C. "Wilson passed all three levels of the CFA examination program in consecutive attempts and earned the right to use the CFA designation."

6. Terry Welch, CFA, is a portfolio manager for Barr Investments. Welch began using Orham Brokers as his sole broker five years ago. Orham's competitive fees and superior trade execution have drawn the attention of Welch's colleagues, many of whom now only use Orham to place trades. In appreciation for the long-standing relationship, Orham offers Welch tickets to a performance of the local symphony, which he accepts. The tickets have a total value of $90. Welch elects not to report the gift to his employer since it does not meet Barr's reportable threshold value of $100. Do Welch's actions with regard to the symphony tickets comply with CFA Institute Standards of Professional Conduct?
   A. Welch has not violated any Standard.
   B. Welch may accept the tickets only with written permission from his employer.
   C. Although his employer's policies do not require Welch to disclose the gift, the Code and Standards require that he do so.

7. Janelle Russ, CFA, is an analyst covering Etrex Company, which is involved in litigation Russ believes could virtually bankrupt the company. In a recent newspaper interview, an Etrex executive said that "we are very near a settlement on that lawsuit that we believe is equitable for all parties." In preparing her next report on Etrex, Russ may:
   A. not mention the settlement because her information comes from a company insider.
   B. not adjust her forecasts for the settlement until the settlement is established as fact.
   C. adjust her forecasts for the settlement, state that this result is based on her opinion, and cite the article that contains the executive's comment.

8. Amy Liu, CFA, and Tom Yang, a CFA candidate, are preparing a research report on Tello Industries. Liu includes quotations about the company's earnings prospects, which she attributes to "investment experts." Yang includes earnings data and balance sheet ratios he obtained from a Standard & Poor's database without citing their source. According to the Standards of Practice:
   A. both analysts have violated the Standards.
   B. neither analyst has violated the Standards.
   C. only one of the analysts has violated the Standards.

9. Danielle Roberts, CFA, a sell-side equity analyst, is finishing a research report on Swift Company. Roberts has owned shares of Swift for over 15 years. Since she began covering Swift as an analyst, her shares have been held in a blind trust account. Roberts does not have the ability to direct trades in the trust and is only informed of the holdings through a general list of securities without individual position values or numbers of shares held. According to the Standards of Professional Conduct, is Roberts required to make any disclosures of her ownership of shares in Swift?
   A. Roberts does not have to make any disclosures as long as the shares are held in the blind trust.
   B. Roberts should disclose her holdings in Swift in her research report, but no disclosure to her employer is required.
   C. Roberts should disclose her holdings in Swift in her research report, as well as to her employer.

10. Robert White is a client of Song Investments, a full-service brokerage firm that produces its own investment research. A firm analyst changes her recommendation from "Buy" to "Sell" on one of the stocks that White holds in his portfolio and sends an e-mail to all firm clients, including White, informing them of the investment recommendation change. White phones John Smith, CFA, his broker at Song Investments, and asks him to buy more of all stocks that White holds in his account with the firm. Smith executes the order. With respect to fair dealing, Smith:
    A. did not violate the Standards because his firm had already sent White an e-mail about the change in recommendation and the order is unsolicited.
    B. did not violate the Standards because it is the analyst's responsibility to communicate changes in her investment recommendations.
    C. violated the Standards because he should have informed White of the change of investment recommendation from buy to sell prior to accepting the order.

11. Roger Anthony, CFA, is an investment adviser. Last year, he advised three of his clients to invest in Abco stock. All three purchased the stock and continue to own it. Anthony inherits more than $1,000,000 of Abco stock. Anthony discloses the receipt of the stock to his supervisor, but takes no further action. Has Anthony complied with the Standards of Professional Conduct?
    A. Yes, Anthony has fulfilled the requirements of the Standard regarding the disclosure of a potential conflict of interest.
    B. No, Anthony must also disclose his position in Abco to his clients.
    C. No, Anthony should transfer management of these clients' portfolios to another advisor.

12. Janet Kelley, CFA, and Verne Gordon, CFA, are both technology analysts. Kelley and Gordon attend a meeting with DM Microchips, where DM's management discusses possible closure of one of DM's manufacturing plants. Which of the following statements is the *most* accurate?
    A. Kelley and Gordon should urge full public disclosure of the plant closure information.
    B. Kelley and Gordon are free to disclose information covered in the meeting to their clients.
    C. The effect on DM's stock price is indeterminate, thus this information is not considered material nonpublic information.

13. Brian Lewis, CFA, is a sales associate for Kite Brothers. Kite Brothers compensates sales associates for referring clients to other units of the company. Lewis recommends that a client transfer his personal accounts to the retail area of Kite Brothers. He gives the client supporting documentation that Kite Brothers is a leader in the retail brokerage industry with a competitive fee structure. The client reviews the material and decides to move his personal accounts to Kite Brothers. Has Lewis violated the Standards of Professional Conduct?
    A. No, because Lewis was participating in a legitimate incentive program established by his employer.
    B. Yes, because Lewis is required to refuse any compensation arrangement that creates a conflict of interest with his clients.
    C. Yes, because Lewis did not disclose the compensation he earned for the referral to another department within Kite Brothers.

14. According to the GIPS fundamentals of compliance, under the requirements regarding the definition of the firm, what is the correct procedure for what type of assets are to be included in "total firm assets"?
    A. Non-fee paying accounts can be excluded from total firm assets.
    B. Total firm assets include discretionary and non-discretionary assets, and include both fee-paying and non-fee paying accounts.
    C. Total firm assets include both fee-paying and non-fee-paying accounts, but composites containing non-discretionary assets may be excluded from total firm assets.

15. Ron Brenner, CFA, manages portfolios for individuals. One of his clients, John Perlman, offers Brenner several inducements above those provided by his employer to motivate superior future performance in managing his portfolio. Brenner notifies his manager via e-mail about the terms of this offer, and his employer grants permission. According to the Standard on additional compensation arrangements, Brenner:
    A. must notify "all parties involved," which includes his other clients.
    B. has taken all the actions required to accept the arrangement.
    C. should decline this arrangement because it could cause partiality in the handling of other client accounts.

16. Nancy Wiley, CFA, suspects that one of her clients is involved in illegal money-laundering activity, and may have large amounts of unreported income. To comply with the Code and Standards, Wiley's *best* course of action is to:
    A. report the suspected activity to the authorities, as required by law.
    B. report the activity and dissociate from managing that client's account.
    C. inform her supervisor, check with her firm's compliance department and possibly outside counsel, and allow her employer to determine the proper steps to take.

17. With respect to a member's activities when leaving a firm, under the Code and Standards, it is *least likely* that:
    A. using knowledge of client names after leaving the firm is permissible.
    B. it is acceptable to take firm records or work performed on the employer's behalf, if the employer grants permission.
    C. the employee's skills and knowledge obtained while employed are considered confidential or privileged information of the employer.

18. Roger Smith, CFA, manages a retirement account for his father-in-law. Smith notices that a stock his father-in-law owns has been downgraded by his firm's research department. Smith places a "sell" order for the entire position in that stock for three clients' accounts, one of which belongs to his father-in-law. According to the CFA Institute Standards of Professional Conduct, Smith:
    A. has violated the Standards because he has beneficial ownership in the account.
    B. has not violated any Standard because his father-in-law's account should be treated like any other firm account.
    C. has violated the Standards by entering a transaction before all clients have had adequate opportunity to act on the recommendation.

Questions 19 through 32 relate to Quantitative Methods. (21 minutes)

19. A study finds that stocks with low price-to-book-value ratios, using end-of-year stock prices and book values per share, have positive abnormal returns in January on average. This study *most likely* suffers from:
    A. look-ahead bias.
    B. time-period bias.
    C. sample selection bias.

20. George Hutchins, CFA, would like to perform a paired comparisons test on returns for the stocks of two real estate investment trusts. The test statistic that Hutchins should select for the paired comparisons test is the:
    A. t-statistic.
    B. F-statistic.
    C. Chi-square statistic.

21. Merle Newman is forecasting unit demand of Tilt Company, a producer of specialty pinball machines. Newman lists his results in the following table:

Unit Forecast	*Probability Function*
500	0.20
1,000	0.20
1,500	0.20
2,000	0.20
2,500	0.20

The probability that Tilt Company unit demand will fall in the range of 1,000 to 2,000 units, inclusive, is *closest* to:
A. 20%.
B. 60%.
C. 80%.

22. The joint probability distribution for the return of two retail stocks, A-Marts and Shops R Us, is provided below.

Retail Scenario	*Probability*	*Return for A-Marts*	*Return for Shops R Us*
Good	0.35	0.20	0.10
Average	0.50	0.04	0.02
Poor	0.15	–0.20	–0.10

The covariance between returns for A-Marts and Shops R Us is:
A. less than 0.
B. at least 0, but less than 0.01.
C. greater than 0.01.

23. Norton Hurro, CFA, is the portfolio manager for the Universe Fund. The market value of the Universe Fund was $10 million at the beginning of year 1. The following events took place in the Universe Fund over the past two years:

- Dividends totaling $500,000 were paid to shareholders at the end of year 1.
- Withdrawals totaling $2 million were made by shareholders at the end of year 1.
- The rate of return on the Universe Fund in year 1 was 10.0%.
- Dividends totaling $400,000 were paid to shareholders at the end of year 2.
- The year 2 year-end market value of the Universe Fund was $9 million.
- The rate of return on the Universe Fund in year 2 was 11.5%.
- No dividends were reinvested by the shareholders.

The money-weighted return on the Universe Fund over the 2-year period is:
A. between 9.5% and 10.0%.
B. between 10.0% and 10.5%.
C. between 10.5% and 11.0%.

24. Mathias Lacros, CFA, owns an emerging market portfolio of 20 stocks with returns that are non-normally distributed. One of Lacros's clients asks him to estimate the range within which at least 75% of the annual returns will lie. To answer his client's question, Lacros should use:
A. the central limit theorem.
B. Chebyshev's inequality.
C. Roy's safety-first ratio.

25. Jacques Welch, security analyst for Z-Investments, selects stocks based on a proprietary stock screen. Returns on stocks satisfying Welch's stock screen are assumed to be normally distributed with the following characteristics:

- Mean annual return = 10%
- Standard deviation = 5%

The probability that a randomly selected stock which satisfies the stock screen will lose money next year is *closest* to:
A. 2.5%.
B. 5.0%.
C. 10.0%.

26. VCI, a venture capital firm, tests a hypothesis on venture capital mean rates of return. The results of their tests lead VCI to not reject the null hypothesis that the population mean rate of return for venture capital investments equals 15%. Tests were conducted over a period during which the market return was 10%. The *best* interpretation of this result is:
    A. most sampled venture capital investments earned a return greater than the market return.
    B. the average rate of return for the 100 sampled venture capital investments equaled 15%.
    C. the sampled average rate of return for venture capital investments did not provide sufficient evidence to contradict the null hypothesis.

27. The probability that the economy will enter a recession after the Federal Reserve increases the federal funds target rate is 60%, and the probability that the economy will enter a recession if the Federal Reserve does not increase the federal funds target rate is 10%. The unconditional probability that the economy will fall into recession is determined using the:
    A. total probability rule.
    B. addition rule for probabilities.
    C. multiplication rule for probabilities.

28. Assumptions of technical analysis are *least likely* to include that:
    A. security prices exhibit persistent trends.
    B. current security prices reflect all available information.
    C. both rational and irrational behavior drive supply and demand.

29. Jacob Monroe, CFA, is forecasting the price of a stock one year from now and compiles a cumulative distribution function of his estimated probabilities for the possible stock values:

Stock Price	*Cumulative Distribution Function*
$5	1%
$10	11%
$15	26%
$20	46%
$25	66%
$30	81%
$35	88%
$40	93%
$45	96%
$50	98%

Based on the table above, Monroe estimates that the stock price one year from now:

A. is most likely to be $50.
B. has an 88% probability of being $35 or less.
C. has a 66% probability of being $25 or greater.

30. Jack Long, CFA, is evaluating the retirement account of John Smith. Smith currently has $500,000 and will retire in 12 years. Smith plans to contribute $12,700 per year. If Smith needs $2 million at retirement, the return required is *closest* to:

A. 10%.
B. 11%.
C. 12%.

31. David Hick, CFA, is reviewing the monthly performance of his fund over the past 20 years. The mean performance was 11.7% with a standard deviation of 21.4%. The return distribution is shown graphically below.

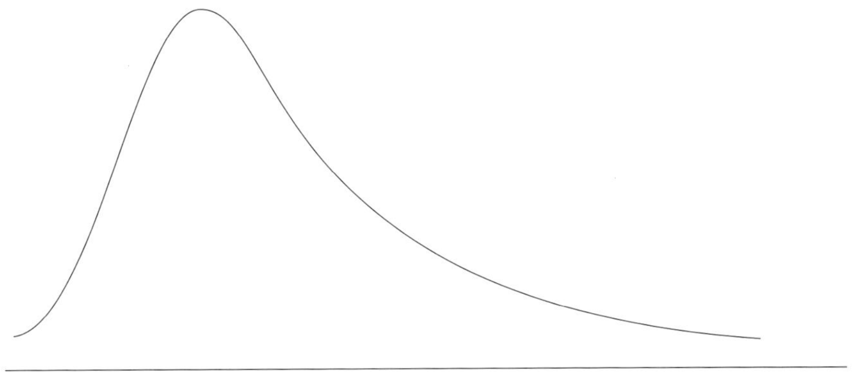

Indicate the relationship of the mean, median, and mode in the above distribution.
A. Mean < median < mode.
B. Mean < median > mode.
C. Mean > median > mode.

32. The bond-equivalent yield on a semiannual coupon bond is 8.5%. The effective annual yield on the bond is:
A. equal to 8.5%.
B. less than 8.5%.
C. greater than 8.5%.

Questions 33 through 44 relate to Economics. (18 minutes)

33. A profit-maximizing firm in short-run equilibrium sells 300 units, has total revenue of 12,000, and marginal revenue of 25. It is *most likely* that this firm:
A. earns an economic profit.
B. faces a perfectly elastic demand curve.
C. should invest in productive capacity to increase profits.

34. With respect to the IS-LM model, which of the following factors is held constant when combining the IS and LM curves to generate the aggregate demand curve?
A. Price level.
B. Real money supply.
C. Nominal money supply.

35. Placing a tariff on imports of a good is *most likely* to decrease:
A. producer surplus for domestic producers of the good.
B. quantity of the good supplied by domestic producers.
C. quantity of the good demanded in the domestic market.

36. A country's statistical bureau reports a GDP deflator of 106.5. An analyst should interpret this statistic to mean that:
A. the annual inflation rate is 6.5%.
B. nominal GDP is 6.5% greater than real GDP.
C. nominal GDP has increased at a 6.5% annual rate.

37. An economist finds the following characteristics for the market for two products, S and T:

Product	*Firm's Pricing Power*	*Concentration Ratio*
S	Considerable	High
T	Some	Low

Based on the above characteristics, the economist could conclude that the industry for Product S is:
A. an oligopoly and the industry for Product T is also an oligopoly.
B. an oligopoly and the industry for Product T is monopolistic competition.
C. monopolistic competition and the industry for product T is an oligopoly.

38. Which of the following statements about the elasticities and absorption approaches to explaining the impact of exchange rate changes on trade deficits is *most accurate*?
A. Both the elasticities and absorption approaches consider trade and capital flows.
B. Under the elasticities approach, currency depreciation will result in greater improvement in the trade deficit when either import or export demand becomes more elastic.
C. Under the absorption approach, depreciation of the domestic currency will improve a trade deficit if it increases national expenditures relative to income.

39. The difference in production outcomes between monopolistic firms and purely competitive firms is *best* explained by the fact that:
A. the profit maximizing output level for monopolists occurs at lower levels of production than for purely competitive firms.
B. monopolists maximize profits by setting output such that marginal revenue exceeds marginal cost.
C. monopolists maximize profits by setting output such that marginal revenue is maximized.

40. At a base period, the nominal exchange rate for Potter (PTR) and Balt (BAL) is 2.50 PTR/BAL. Two years later, if the nominal exchange rate is 3.00 PTR/BAL, the Potter CPI is 120, and the Balt CPI is 110:
A. the real PTR/BAL exchange rate has increased.
B. the purchasing power of one PTR in terms of Balt goods has increased.
C. exports from Potter to Balt have become relatively more expensive to residents of Balt.

41. If there is an increase in the quantity of money at full employment, the long-run effects will *most likely* be:
A. an increase in the price level and a decrease in real GDP.
B. an increase in the price level and no effect on real GDP.
C. no effect on the price level and no effect on real GDP.

42. The government of Wallvania is evaluating the impact of a new tax on automobiles that will be levied on manufacturers. Research on the auto market in Wallvania shows that supply is more elastic than demand. Which of the following statements is *most* accurate?
A. Auto manufacturers will bear the entire tax burden.
B. Consumers will bear a greater portion of the tax burden.
C. Auto manufacturers will bear a greater portion of the tax burden.

43. The Federal Reserve has decided to increase the federal funds rate (the interest rate that banks charge each other for overnight loans). To implement this policy, the Federal Reserve will *most likely*:
A. sell government securities in the open market.
B. increase currency exchange rates (cause domestic currency to appreciate).
C. set a lower price on Treasury bills and notes that it is auctioning.

44. Rusty Brown worked at a food processing plant. In a move to reduce costs, the plant automated the production line where Brown worked. Brown was laid off because he was not adequately trained to work the new equipment. Gilda Gold was the bookkeeper for a coal mine that was closed because it could not meet safety standards. Which type of unemployment is illustrated by each worker?
A. Brown and Gold are both examples of frictional unemployment.
B. Brown is an example of structural unemployment and Gold is an example of cyclical unemployment.
C. Brown is an example of structural unemployment and Gold is an example of frictional unemployment.

Questions 45 through 68 relate to Financial Reporting and Analysis. (36 minutes)

45. The main objectives of an independent audit are to:
    A. determine whether employees of the entity comply with established policies and to verify inventory amounts and cash balances.
    B. selectively examine evidence supporting the amounts and disclosures in the financial statements and to prepare the necessary financial statements for reporting purposes.
    C. determine whether the financial statements were prepared in accordance with generally accepted accounting principles and to selectively examine evidence supporting the amounts and disclosures in the financial statements.

46. Under U.S. GAAP, dividends paid to shareholders should be classified in the cash flow statement as:
    A. operating activity.
    B. financing activity.
    C. investing activity.

47. Joe's Supermarket has been experiencing rising product prices, while quantities sold have remained stable. The company uses the LIFO method to account for its inventory. If the company had used the FIFO method, what impact would it have had on the company's working capital?
    A. Higher working capital balance.
    B. Lower working capital balance.
    C. No impact on working capital.

48. Gravel Inc. purchased a large crane to improve the production efficiency of its roadway construction division. The cost of the machine was $550,000 and it has a useful life of ten years, at which point the equipment will have a salvage value of $50,000. Depreciation expense for the second year of the asset's life using the double declining balance method is *closest* to:
    A. $50,000.
    B. $88,000.
    C. $110,000.

49. On January 1, National Beverage Vending had 100,000 shares of common stock issued and outstanding. On June 1, the company repurchased 20,000 shares at $12 per share. On August 1, the common stock was split 2 for 1. Weighted average shares outstanding for the year are *closest* to:
    A. 83,333.
    B. 93,333.
    C. 176,667.

50. A food wholesale company has an investment portfolio of frequently traded securities and longer-term investments that are available for sale. U.S. GAAP requires unrealized gains and losses on the longer-term investments to be reported:
A. in non-operating income.
B. in a separate section following net income.
C. as other comprehensive income on the statement of changes in owners' equity.

51. Under U.S. GAAP, costs of a 2-year final testing program for a new drug would be:
A. measured at actual cost as they occur and recorded as expenses on the income statement.
B. measured at the present value of expected costs for the 2-year program and capitalized as an intangible asset.
C. estimated and expensed in equal amounts over the next two years.

52. Gus Swenson, CFA, develops a new method for accelerated depreciation that he believes will reflect economic reality for some firms better than existing methods. Which of the following organizations is *most likely* to determine whether firms may adopt Swenson's method?
A. Securities and Exchange Commission.
B. International Accounting Standards Board.
C. International Organization of Securities Commissions.

53. Which of these intangible assets is *most likely* to be amortized?
A. Purchased patent that will expire in the current period.
B. Purchased franchise right with a useful life of two years.
C. Internally developed trademark with a useful life of 20 years.

54. For an analyst, disclosures about financing liabilities in the financial statement footnotes and management's commentary would be *most useful* in determining the:
A. firm's leverage.
B. market value of the firm's outstanding debt.
C. timing and amount of future financing cash flows.

55. Which of the following is *most likely* reported as a financing activity on the cash flow statement?
A. Conversion of debt to equity.
B. Repayment of long-term debt.
C. Acquisition of a company through the assumption of its liabilities.

56. Balance sheet changes *most likely* to be consistent with a decrease in cash of $10,000 are a(n):
    A. increase in accounts payable of $3,000 and an increase in inventories of $13,000.
    B. decrease in notes payable of $12,000 and an increase in marketable securities of $2,000.
    C. increase in accounts receivable of $14,000 and a decrease in retained earnings of $4,000.

57. Carlton Corp., a large manufacturing company, is currently negotiating a new contract with its unionized employees. Which of the following accounting red flags would potentially indicate manipulation to improve the company's bargaining position?
    A. Deferral of expenses.
    B. LIFO liquidation at year-end.
    C. Not capitalizing certain expenses.

58. For a firm that uses debt financing, the difference between free cash flow to the firm and free cash flow to equity is equal to:
    A. interest expense × (1 – tax rate).
    B. interest expense + net borrowing.
    C. interest expense × (1 – tax rate) – net borrowing.

59. Red Company acquired Raider Incorporated at the end of last year. As a part of the acquisition, Red recognized goodwill of $75,000. At the end of this year, the following data was compiled:

Fair value of Red Company	$600,000
Fair value of Raider Incorporated	$400,000
Carrying value of Red Company	$540,000
Carrying value of Raider Incorporated	$385,000*
*including goodwill	

According to U.S GAAP, Red Company should test for goodwill impairment and recognize:
    A. a $15,000 loss.
    B. a $60,000 gain.
    C. no gain or loss.

60. Dot Corporation uses accelerated depreciation for tax purposes and straight-line depreciation for financial reporting. The company has a large cash position which is invested in tax-free municipal bonds. With regard to Dot's financial statements and tax reporting:
    A. both the interest income and the depreciation method will necessitate the use of a valuation allowance account.
    B. the interest income will result in a deferred tax asset and the depreciation method will result in a deferred tax liability.
    C. the depreciation expense causes a temporary difference between income tax expense and taxes payable, and the interest income creates a permanent difference.

61. Items on a balance sheet that are expected to provide future economic benefits and are a result of previous transactions are classified as:
    A. assets.
    B. liabilities.
    C. stockholders' equity.

62. A firm's statement of changes in equity shows an increase in shareholders' equity of $7 million. Retained earnings were $6 million over the reporting period. The difference of $1 million *most likely* results from:
    A. receiving dividends.
    B. issuing common stock.
    C. realizing a gain on available-for-sale securities.

63. When screening for potential equity investments, if two of the financial analysis criteria used in the screen are dependent, this will tend to:
    A. increase the number of stocks that pass the screen.
    B. decrease the number of stocks that pass the screen.
    C. have no predictable effect on the number of stocks that pass the screen.

64. Compared to a lessee that uses finance (capital) leases, a lessee that uses operating leases will have a lower:
    A. return on assets.
    B. interest coverage ratio.
    C. debt-to-equity ratio.

65. Rustic Company has recognized an impairment loss on the value of inventory. If the inventory's value subsequently recovers, under which accounting standards may Rustic revalue the inventory upward and recognize a gain?
    A. Neither IFRS nor U.S. GAAP allows a recovery in inventory value to be recognized as a gain.
    B. IFRS allows a recovery in inventory value to be recognized as a gain, but U.S. GAAP does not.
    C. U.S. GAAP allows a recovery in inventory value to be recognized as a gain, but IFRS does not.

66. Spiral Corporation uses a periodic inventory system and the LIFO inventory cost flow assumption, and provided the following information for the period just ended.

	Units	*Unit Cost*	*Total Cost*
Beginning inventory	1,300	$50	$65,000
First purchase	500	$48	$24,000
Second purchase	900	$46	$41,400
Total available	2,700		$130,400
Sold	2,100		

If Spiral had used the FIFO inventory cost flow assumption, its ending inventory would be:
A. $2,400 lower.
B. $1,600 higher.
C. $3,000 higher.

67. Below are selected data from Denton Corporation's 20X7 and 20X8 financial statements:

	20X7	20X8
Preferred stock, 8%, $100 par, nonconvertible	$12.5 million	$12.5 million
Common stock, $10 par	$3 million	$4 million
Additional paid-in-capital, common stock	$30 million	$40 million
Retained earnings	$75 million	$88 million
Treasury stock, at cost	$4 million	$4 million
Net income	$9 million	$14 million

Denton's return on common equity for 20X8 is *closest* to:
A. 10.9%.
B. 11.2%.
C. 12.1%.

68. Bivac Corp. has been experiencing a declining return on equity over the past few years. Selected financial statement ratios for Bivac appear below:

	Prior Year	Current Year
Tax Burden	0.60	0.62
Interest Burden	0.80	0.81
EBIT Margin	0.26	0.26
Asset Turnover	1.06	1.06
ROE	0.15	0.14

What is the *most likely* reason for the decline in Bivac's ROE?
A. Leverage has declined.
B. The tax rate has increased.
C. Net profit margin has declined.

Questions 69 through 78 relate to Corporate Finance. (15 minutes)

69. Companies that can only raise a limited amount of funds to invest in projects must use:
A. capital rationing.
B. project sequencing.
C. capital preservation.

70. Which of the following share repurchase methods is *most likely* to be used in a "greenmail" takeover defense?
A. Tender offer.
B. Direct negotiation.
C. Purchase in the market.

71. Which of the following statements is *most* accurate regarding the net present value (NPV) and internal rate of return (IRR) capital budgeting methods?
A. NPV assumes that cash flows can be reinvested at the project's IRR.
B. IRR assumes the cash flows are reinvested at the project's cost of capital.
C. NPV assumes the cash flows can be reinvested at the project's cost of capital.

72. Good corporate governance practices seek to ensure that the:
A. board of directors protects management interests.
B. firm acts lawfully and ethically in dealings with shareholders.
C. board acts in concert with the firm's executives to ensure cohesive management.

73. An analyst is studying the tax exposures and capital structures of Alpha Corporation and Beta Corporation. Both companies have equivalent weights of debt and equity in their capital structures. Pretax component costs of capital are the same for both companies. Alpha has total capital of $850 million while Beta has total capital of $370 million. The marginal tax rates for Alpha and Beta are 35% and 40%, respectively. Which of the following statements regarding Alpha and Beta is *least* accurate?
   A. Beta Corporation has a lower WACC than Alpha Corporation.
   B. An increase in Alpha Corporation's tax rate would decrease its WACC.
   C. A tax rate change will affect Alpha Corporation's cost of equity more than Beta Corporation.

74. Allen Company's cost of preferred equity is 6.25%. The preferred pays a $2.50 dividend and has a par value of $50. The price of Allen's preferred equity is *closest* to:
   A. $30 per share.
   B. $40 per share.
   C. $50 per share.

75. Regarding shareholder voting, interests of shareowners are *least likely* served by a firm that:
   A. requires attendance at annual meetings in order to vote shares.
   B. has a third party tabulate votes and requires an audit of the tabulation.
   C. provides for cumulative voting.

76. An analyst has calculated the following statistics for Company X and Company Y.

	Company X		*Company Y*	
	Year 1	*Year 2*	*Year 1*	*Year 2*
Number of days of inventory	18	22	33	24
Number of days of receivables	14	16	14	12
Number of days of payables	19	20	18	20

The net operating cycle for:
   A. Company Y was 16 days in year 2, an improvement in liquidity compared to year 1.
   B. Company Y was 36 days in year 2, a decline in liquidity compared to year 1.
   C. Company X was 18 days in year 2, an improvement in liquidity compared to year 1.

77. A portfolio manager buys $1 million of U.S. Treasury bills maturing in 90 days at a price of $990,390 and discount rate of 3.8%. The portfolio also includes the following investments:

- Bank commercial paper maturing in 90 days with a bond equivalent yield of 4.34% and a market value of $100,000.
- Bank certificates of deposit maturing in six months with a bond equivalent yield of 4.84% and a market value of $200,000.

The bond-equivalent yield of a comparable benchmark portfolio is 4.0%. Including the Treasury bill purchase, the manager's portfolio is:
A. outperforming the benchmark.
B. underperforming the benchmark.
C. performing in line with the benchmark.

78. The net present value method of evaluating projects is *most likely* to be chosen instead of the payback period method by firms that are:
A. privately held.
B. larger than average.
C. located in European countries.

Questions 79 through 84 relate to Portfolio Management. (9 minutes)

79. In a case where a client's capacity to bear risk is significantly greater than the client's expressed willingness to bear risk, the *most* appropriate action for a financial advisor is to:
A. counsel the client and attempt to change his attitude towards risk.
B. attempt to educate the client about investment risk and correct any misconceptions.
C. base the assessment of risk tolerance in the IPS on the client's willingness to bear risk.

80. The theoretical market portfolio used to form the Capital Market Line is a(n):
A. market weighted portfolio of all risky assets.
B. market weighted portfolio of all stocks and bonds.
C. equal weighted portfolio of all risky assets available to an investor.

81. Thomas Green, CFA, has forecast the returns for three stocks and plotted these expected returns against the security market line (SML). Bacia Company has a beta of 0.8 and plots above the SML. Zyrox, Inc. has a beta of 1.0 and plots below the SML. Tisher Industries has a beta of 1.2 and plots on the SML. What should Green conclude about the valuation of these stocks?
A. Bacia is overvalued.
B. Zyrox is overvalued.
C. Tisher is overvalued.

82. Historically, returns on major asset classes have exhibited:
A. positive skewness and negative excess kurtosis.
B. negative skewness and positive excess kurtosis.
C. negative skewness and negative excess kurtosis.

83. Patrick Manning owns stock in Lumber Providers with a variance of returns equal to 16%. Manning is considering the addition of Smithson Homebuilders to his portfolio. The variance of returns for Smithson equals 25%, and its correlation of returns with Lumber equals –0.60. The covariance of returns between Lumber and Smithson is *closest* to:
A. –15.0.
B. –0.024.
C. –0.120.

84. A portfolio manager for Klein Capital Management has been slowly increasing the number of stocks in his portfolio randomly over the last five years. Currently, the portfolio contains 20 stocks. Over time, what has *most likely* happened to the risk of the portfolio if macroeconomic variables have remained steady?
A. Unsystematic risk has been decreasing.
B. Systematic risk has been decreasing.
C. Both systematic and unsystematic risk remain at average levels.

Questions 85 through 96 relate to Equity Investments. (18 minutes)

85. Which of the following is *most accurate* regarding the relationship between operational efficiency and informational efficiency?
A. Operational efficiency contributes to informational efficiency.
B. Informational efficiency is independent of operational efficiency.
C. There is a trade-off between operational efficiency and informational efficiency.

86. From the investor's point of view, a firm's preference shares have the *most* risk if they are:
A. putable and non-callable.
B. cumulative and non-putable.
C. callable and non-cumulative.

87. Yong Kim, CFA, buys a preferred stock that has a 6% dividend yield (defined as the ratio of the preferred dividend to the market price of the preferred stock). One year later, Kim sells the stock when it is selling at a 5% dividend yield. The preferred stock pays a fixed annual dividend, which Kim received right before selling. What rate of return did Kim realize on his investment?
A. 14%.
B. 20%.
C. 26%.

88. Roger Templeton, CFA, an analyst for Bridgetown Capital Management, is studying past market data to identify risk factors that produce anomalous returns. He tests monthly data on each of 60 financial and economic variables over a 15-year period to find which ones are related to stock index returns. Templeton identifies three variables that show statistically significant relationships with equity returns at a 95% confidence level. What is the *most likely* reason why Bridgetown's management should be skeptical of the anomalies Templeton has identified? The results suffer from:
   A. data mining bias.
   B. survivorship bias.
   C. small sample bias.

89. A given percentage change in one of the 30 stocks in the Dow Jones Industrial Average (DJIA) will have the greatest impact on the DJIA for which index stock?
   A. The one whose total equity has the highest market value.
   B. The one whose stock trades at the highest dollar price per share.
   C. The one having the greatest amount of equity in its capital structure.

90. A securities exchange is structured as a call market. On that exchange, a stock would trade at:
   A. any time the market is open.
   B. one negotiated price that clears the market.
   C. prices set by auction or by dealer bid-ask quotes.

91. At the end of the last 12-month period, Romano's Italian Foods had net income of $16.68 million and equity of $115 million. Romano's declared a $7.5 million dividend for the year. Using internally generated funds, Romano's can grow its equity by approximately:
   A. 8.0% per year.
   B. 10.0% per year.
   C. 14.5% per year.

92. A market researcher is analyzing the efficiency of the Oceania Securities Exchange (OSE). Market prices appear to incorporate all prior price and volume information in a timely manner but are slow to incorporate the true value impact of earnings surprises. The researcher determines that specialists on the floor of the OSE consistently earn positive risk-adjusted returns on average. Which of the three forms of the Efficient Market Hypothesis *best* describes the OSE market?
   A. Weak-form efficient.
   B. Strong-form efficient.
   C. Semistrong-form efficient.

93. Rock Inc. maintains a policy of paying 30% of earnings to its investors in the form of dividends. Rock is expected to generate a return on equity of 9.3%. Rock's beta is 1.5. The equity risk premium is 6% and U.S. Treasury notes are yielding 3%. Rock's required rate of return is *closest* to:
A. 9.0%.
B. 9.3%.
C. 12.0%.

94. Industry rotation is *best* described as the:
A. adjusting the industry weights in a portfolio based on the current stage of the business cycle.
B. recommended practice of periodically changing the industries that investment analysts are assigned to cover.
C. long-term trend of talented managers and employees exiting mature and declining industries and entering embryonic and growth industries.

95. Jerry Slotz enters an exchange-traded contract that obligates him to purchase a specific amount of an asset on a future date. The contract is *most likely* a(n):
A. option contract.
B. futures contract.
C. forward contract.

96. Jim Boo, CFA, is analyzing Justin Corp., a maker of home appliances. Boo's research provides the following facts:

- Justin's stock price is $60 per share.
- Expected growth rate of dividends is 5%.
- Expected retention ratio is 60%.
- Required rate of return is 10%.

Justin's expected price to earnings ratio (P_0/E_1) is *closest* to:
A. 8.0x.
B. 10.0x.
C. 12.0x.

Questions 97 through 110 relate to Fixed Income. (21 minutes)

97. Omega Corp. has outstanding a $100 million, 9% coupon, callable bond issue that is refund protected until July 1, 20X0. This issue:
A. may not be called until July 1, 20X0.
B. currently may be redeemed with funds from general operations.
C. may only be redeemed if it is refunded by an issue with a lower cost.

98. The current price of a \$1,000 par value, 6-year, 4.2% semiannual coupon bond is \$958.97. The bond's price value of a basis point is *closest* to:
A. \$0.50.
B. \$4.20.
C. \$5.01.

99. Alice Perry, CFA, and Bob Klein, CFA, are discussing the process for valuing a bond. Perry states that the three major steps in valuing a bond are to estimate the cash flows, determine the appropriate discount rate, and compute the present value of the cash flows. Klein adds that when estimating a bond's cash flows, only the timing and amount of coupon payments need to be estimated. Are Perry and Klein correct regarding the process for valuing a bond?
A. Both of these statements are accurate.
B. Neither of these statements is accurate.
C. Only one of these statements is accurate.

100. Bond X and Bond Y were issued at a premium to par value three years ago. Bond X matures in five years, and Bond Y matures in ten years. Both bonds carry the same credit rating. Bond X has a coupon of 7.25%, and Bond Y has a coupon of 8.00%. If the yield to maturity for both bonds is 7.60% today:
A. both bonds are priced at a premium.
B. Bond X is priced at a premium, and Bond Y is priced at a discount.
C. Bond X is priced at a discount, and Bond Y is priced at a premium

101. Debt securities that are combined with derivatives are referred to as:
A. secured bonds.
B. structured notes.
C. bankers acceptances.

102. Rob Pirate is considering investing in a subordinated tranche in a collateralized mortgage obligation (CMO). If Pirate wishes to measure his interest rate risk for this debt security, which measure would be *most* appropriate?
A. Modified duration.
B. Effective duration.
C. Effective convexity.

103. Mark Davidson and James Case are bond traders at a large fixed-income investment firm. Both Davidson and Case have developed bond valuation models for bonds with embedded options. Using their respective models, the traders have calculated the price of BMC Corp.'s callable and putable bonds. Davidson uses a yield volatility assumption of 23%, while Case uses an assumption of 31%. Other than the volatility assumption, the traders use identical inputs for the models. Which of the following *best* summarizes the output of the two valuation models?
A. Davidson's model will calculate a lower value for the call option and a lower value for the putable bond.
B. Case's model will calculate a higher value for the call option and a lower value for the putable bond.
C. Davidson's model will calculate a lower value for the put option and a lower value for the callable bond.

104. Explaining the shape of the yield curve, fixed income securities analyst Thomas Smith states that bond investors require a risk premium to hold longer-term bonds. Smith is describing the:
A. pure expectations theory.
B. liquidity preference theory.
C. market segmentation theory.

105. Laura Mack, CFA, is considering purchasing two Treasury securities. The first is the 7-year on-the-run Treasury issued last week that has a coupon rate of 5%. The second is a 7-year off-the-run Treasury that was issued two months ago and has a coupon rate of 4.75%. The on-the-run issue has:
A. higher reinvestment risk because of its higher coupon rate.
B. higher interest rate risk because of its higher coupon rate.
C. the same interest rate risk as the off-the-run issue.

106. An investor wants to take advantage of the 5-year spot rate, currently at a level of 4.0%. Unfortunately, the investor just invested all of his funds in a 2-year bond with a yield of 3.2%. The investor contacts his broker, who tells him that in two years he can purchase a 3-year bond and end up with the same return currently offered on the 5-year bond. What 3-year forward rate beginning two years from now will allow the investor to earn a return equivalent to the 5-year spot rate?
A. 3.5%.
B. 4.5%.
C. 5.6%.

107. Consider a 10-year, 6% coupon, $1,000 par value bond, paying annual coupons, with a 10% yield to maturity. The change in the bond price resulting from a 400 basis point increase in yield is *closest* to:
A. $170.
B. $480.
C. $1,160.

108. The return impact of a 25 basis point widening in yield spread for an option-free bond is greatest if it has a duration of:
A. 4 and convexity of 24.
B. 5 and convexity of 32.
C. 6 and convexity of 90.

109. Allison Coleman, CFA, owns a bond portfolio that includes Bond X, a callable bond with ten years to maturity that is callable at any time beginning one year from today. Coleman's portfolio also includes Bond Y, a noncallable security with ten years to maturity that carries the same credit rating as Bond X. Coleman expects interest rates to decrease steadily over the next few years. Based on this assumption, Coleman should expect that:
A. Bond Y will experience a larger decrease in value than Bond X.
B. Bond X will benefit from positive convexity as rates decline.
C. the option embedded in Bond X will increase in value.

110. Jefferson Blake, CFA, believes there is a good opportunity to purchase an option-free 4% annual pay bond with three years left until maturity, a zero-volatility spread of 40 basis points, and a par value of $1,000. Blake observes that 1-year, 2-year, and 3-year Treasury STRIP rates are currently 4.0%, 4.5%, and 4.75%, respectively. The maximum price Blake should be willing to pay for the bond is *closest* to:
A. $940.
B. $970.
C. $980.

Questions 111 through 116 relate to Derivatives. (9 minutes)

111. For an American-style call option with an exercise price of €30 on a stock trading at €34, the theoretical minimum value prior to expiration is:
A. equal to the theoretical minimum value of an otherwise identical European call.
B. less than the theoretical minimum value of an otherwise identical European call.
C. greater than the theoretical minimum value of an otherwise identical European call.

112. In futures markets, the primary role of the clearinghouse is to:
A. prevent arbitrage and enforce federal regulations.
B. act as guarantor to both sides of a futures trade.
C. reduce transaction costs by making contract prices public.

113. Janice Grass, CFA, will need to borrow $12 million in an upcoming month. Grass is concerned that the U.S. Federal Reserve will raise interest rates dramatically, so she enters into a 2 × 8 FRA. The FRA is quoted at 6%. LIBOR interest rates on the expiration day of the FRA are presented in the table below.

	Settlement
30-day LIBOR	5.7%
60-day LIBOR	5.8%
120-day LIBOR	5.9%
180-day LIBOR	6.0%
240-day LIBOR	6.1%

The payoff on the FRA is *closest* to:
A. 0.
B. +$2,630.81.
C. –$2,956.39.

114. Lincoln Industrial's current stock price is $64 per share and the company will pay a $0.56 dividend. The 90-day U.S. Treasury bill is yielding 5.3%. Lincoln's 3-month European call option with a strike price of $70 has a premium of $3.50. Based on put-call parity, the value of a Lincoln put option with a strike price of $70 is *closest* to:
A. $8.05.
B. $8.60.
C. $9.15.

115. Peter Black is an options trader for HighSmith Investments. Black trades options on the U.S. and U.K. stock exchanges. Black has been following the price movements of options on two companies: U.S.-based Pacific Chemicals Inc. and U.K.-based Merchant Clothing Co. Black has observed that over the past few days, the prices of put options on Pacific stock have increased, and the prices of call options on Merchant stock have increased. These observations *most likely* suggest that interest rates in:
A. the U.S. have increased and the volatility of Merchant stock has decreased.
B. the U.K. have decreased and the volatility of Pacific stock has increased.
C. the U.S. have decreased and the volatility of Merchant stock has increased.

116. The Pairagain mutual fund has entered into an equity swap with SingleSol, LLC, with a notional principal of $50 million. Pairagain has agreed to pay the quarterly return on the NASDAQ 100 in exchange for a fixed rate of 7.0%. The initial price of the NASDAQ 100 was 1825, and the value at the end of the first quarter, 91 days later, was 1755. The swap uses a 365-day year convention. What is the net payment to be made at the end of the first quarter?
A. SingleSol pays $2,790,411.
B. SingleSol pays $1,917,808.
C. SingleSol pays $872,603.

Questions 117 through 120 relate to Alternative Investments. (6 minutes)

117. If the availability of a physical commodity over the period of a futures contract has value to users of the commodity, the commodity is said to provide:
A. storage yield.
B. collateral yield.
C. convenience yield.

118. A hedge fund started the year with a value of €125 million. At year's end the value before fees is €150 million. The fund charges 2 and 20 with management fees calculated on end-of-year values. Incentive fees are net of management fees and calculated using a 10% hard hurdle rate. Total fees paid for this year are *closest* to:
A. €4.9 million.
B. €5.5 million.
C. €7.4 million.

119. The stage of venture capital investing that involves product development and market research is referred to as the:
A. seed stage.
B. early stage.
C. angel investing stage.

120. Compared to the standard deviation of returns on a repeat sales index for a class of real estate properties, the standard deviation of returns on an appraisal index for the same class of properties is *most likely* to be:
A. lower.
B. higher.
C. the same.

End of Morning Session

Exam 2
Afternoon Session

Topic	Questions	Points
Ethical and Professional Standards	1–18	27
Quantitative Methods	19–32	21
Economics	33–44	18
Financial Reporting and Analysis	45–68	36
Corporate Finance	69–78	15
Portfolio Management	79–84	9
Equity Investments	85–96	18
Fixed Income	97–110	21
Derivatives	111–116	9
Alternative Investments	117–120	6
Total		**180**

Test Answers

1.	A	B	C
2.	A	B	C
3.	A	B	C
4.	A	B	C
5.	A	B	C
6.	A	B	C
7.	A	B	C
8.	A	B	C
9.	A	B	C
10.	A	B	C
11.	A	B	C
12.	A	B	C
13.	A	B	C
14.	A	B	C
15.	A	B	C
16.	A	B	C
17.	A	B	C
18.	A	B	C
19.	A	B	C
20.	A	B	C
21.	A	B	C
22.	A	B	C
23.	A	B	C
24.	A	B	C
25.	A	B	C
26.	A	B	C
27.	A	B	C
28.	A	B	C
29.	A	B	C
30.	A	B	C
31.	A	B	C
32.	A	B	C
33.	A	B	C
34.	A	B	C
35.	A	B	C
36.	A	B	C
37.	A	B	C
38.	A	B	C
39.	A	B	C
40.	A	B	C
41.	A	B	C
42.	A	B	C
43.	A	B	C
44.	A	B	C
45.	A	B	C
46.	A	B	C
47.	A	B	C
48.	A	B	C
49.	A	B	C
50.	A	B	C
51.	A	B	C
52.	A	B	C
53.	A	B	C
54.	A	B	C
55.	A	B	C
56.	A	B	C
57.	A	B	C
58.	A	B	C
59.	A	B	C
60.	A	B	C
61.	A	B	C
62.	A	B	C
63.	A	B	C
64.	A	B	C
65.	A	B	C
66.	A	B	C
67.	A	B	C
68.	A	B	C
69.	A	B	C
70.	A	B	C
71.	A	B	C
72.	A	B	C
73.	A	B	C
74.	A	B	C
75.	A	B	C
76.	A	B	C
77.	A	B	C
78.	A	B	C
79.	A	B	C
80.	A	B	C
81.	A	B	C
82.	A	B	C
83.	A	B	C
84.	A	B	C
85.	A	B	C
86.	A	B	C
87.	A	B	C
88.	A	B	C
89.	A	B	C
90.	A	B	C
91.	A	B	C
92.	A	B	C
93.	A	B	C
94.	A	B	C
95.	A	B	C
96.	A	B	C
97.	A	B	C
98.	A	B	C
99.	A	B	C
100.	A	B	C
101.	A	B	C
102.	A	B	C
103.	A	B	C
104.	A	B	C
105.	A	B	C
106.	A	B	C
107.	A	B	C
108.	A	B	C
109.	A	B	C
110.	A	B	C
111.	A	B	C
112.	A	B	C
113.	A	B	C
114.	A	B	C
115.	A	B	C
116.	A	B	C
117.	A	B	C
118.	A	B	C
119.	A	B	C
120.	A	B	C

Exam 2
Afternoon Session

Questions 1 through 18 relate to Ethical and Professional Standards. (27 minutes)

1. Ronnie Smith is registered to sit for the next CFA Level II exam after failing the exam the past two years. Smith posts the following comment on a popular Internet bulletin board: "I believe CFA Institute is intentionally limiting the number of charterholders to increase its cash flow by continuing to fail candidates." Does Smith's comment violate the Code and Standards?
   A. No.
   B. Yes, because his comment is false.
   C. Yes, because his comment brings CFA Institute into disrepute.

2. Apex Investments has adopted the Global Investment Performance Standards (GIPS)®. The firm had presented performance for a high yield fixed income composite, but discontinued it one year ago. With respect to the discontinued composite, GIPS:
   A. requires that Apex include it on the firm's list of composites.
   B. does not require that Apex include the discontinued composite on the firm's list of composites or make any specific disclosure about it.
   C. requires that Apex include information regarding the discontinued composite in the "Disclosures" section of the presentation, but does not require its inclusion as a composite.

3. Jack Wilson, CFA, a hedge fund manager, takes a large short position in Bonner, Inc. stock. After Wilson establishes his short position, Bonner shares trade down 1.15%. One week later, Bonner shares are trading 3.84% below the initial short price, and Wilson reverses the short position and establishes a short position in shares of the company's competitor, Hatch Company. On a well-known investor message board, Wilson posts a highly critical message about Hatch, which grossly exaggerates problems with a crucial supplier to Hatch. The day after Wilson's message post, Hatch shares fall 0.97% and Wilson reverses the short position. Did Wilson's actions related to Bonner stock and/or Hatch stock violate the CFA Institute Standards of Professional Conduct?
   A. Yes, in both cases.
   B. Only in the case of Hatch.
   C. Only in the case of Bonner.

4. After working 20 years on Wall Street, Jim Gentry, CFA, decides to open his own investment firm on Turtle Island, located in the Caribbean. Turtle Island has securities laws that are much less stringent than U.S. laws or the CFA Institute Standards of Professional Conduct. Many of his U.S.-based clients have agreed to keep Gentry as their portfolio manager and move their assets to his new firm. After a few months of operations, Gentry has encountered several instances in which Turtle Island regulations relieve him of disclosing information to investors that he had been required to disclose while working in New York. According to the CFA Institute Code and Standards, Gentry must adhere to the:
   A. Code and Standards or U.S. law, whichever is more strict.
   B. laws of Turtle Island, but disclose any discrepancies to U.S.-based clients.
   C. Code and Standards because as a charterholder, he need only adhere to the Code and Standards under all circumstances.

5. Rene Green, CFA, uses a statistical model to estimate the intrinsic value of potential investments. Clients are aware of the general model but not its details. Green recently changed the model in an attempt to more accurately price assets. In an e-mail to all of his prospects and clients, Green describes the new model and states that more accurate asset valuations are expected from the new model. Has Green violated the CFA Institute Standards of Professional Conduct?
   A. No, Green's actions are consistent with CFA Institute Standards.
   B. Yes, because he should have notified existing clients before notifying prospects.
   C. Yes, because he suggested that the new model will generate more accurate asset valuations.

6. Thomas Baker recently passed the Level III CFA examination. Baker is reviewing a draft of the firm's marketing material to be distributed after he receives his CFA charter. One passage reads, "Baker is especially proud of the fact that he passed all three Levels of the exam on his first attempts in three consecutive years." Is this statement in compliance with CFA Institute Standards?
   A. Yes, as long as it is a statement of fact.
   B. No, because it implies that Baker has superior ability.
   C. No, because Members or Candidates who passed the exams on their first attempts may not differentiate themselves from those who did not.

7. Jimmy Deininger, CFA, manages several client portfolios. One of his clients offers him use of a cabin in a vacation spot because the client's investment results under Deininger's management have exceeded the client's goals. Deininger discloses the gift to his employer. With reference to the Standards of Practice, Deininger:
   A. has complied with the Standards and may accept the gift.
   B. is not permitted to accept the gift because he does not have permission from his employer.
   C. has appropriately disclosed the gift to his supervisor, but must also disclose it to his other clients.

8. Giselle Holt, CFA, is a portfolio manager in the trust department of State Bank. Holt recently inherited a substantial amount of stock of Brown & Company and accepted a position on the board of directors for TVC Plastics, Inc. Many of the trust clients at the bank hold positions in Brown & Company and in TVC Plastics. According to CFA Institute Standards of Professional Conduct, Holt must disclose:
   A. both the stock ownership and board position to her clients.
   B. the board membership to her clients and the stock ownership to State Bank.
   C. both the stock ownership and board position to her clients and State Bank.

9. Nancy McCoy, CFA, is preparing a report on Gourmet Food Mart. As part of her research, she contacts the company's contractors, suppliers, and competitors. McCoy is told by the CEO of a major produce vendor that he is about to file a lawsuit against Gourmet Food Mart, seeking significant damages. McCoy incorporates this information into her research report, which projects a decline in profitability for Gourmet Food Mart due to the impending litigation. According to the CFA Institute Standards of Professional Conduct, McCoy:
   A. has not violated any Standard.
   B. has violated the Standards by utilizing material nonpublic information.
   C. has violated the Standards by disseminating confidential information.

10. Ron Welch, CFA, manages trust accounts at a regional U.S. bank. Welch was hired four years ago to manage the Craig Family Trust. The investment policy statement for the trust specifies a passive investment strategy of mirroring the risk and return of the S&P 500 Index. Over the past year, Welch over-weighted technology stocks, which allowed the trust portfolio to earn a return 200 basis points above the S&P 500 return with only slightly higher risk. With respect to the Standards concerning suitability and loyalty, prudence, and care, Welch violated:
    A. both of these Standards.
    B. neither of these Standards.
    C. only one of these Standards.

11. Among all analysts who cover Saris Corporation, the consensus earnings estimate for the current period is $2.14. Lee Rutherford, CFA, is convinced that Saris will release earnings substantially above what is anticipated. Rutherford publishes a research report in which he estimates earnings for Saris to be $2.13 per share. In conversations with selected clients, Rutherford mentions his reasons for expecting an announcement of higher earnings. With respect to the Code and Standards:
    A. the conversations do not violate the Standards because the research report is the official document, and that is what Rutherford is supporting.
    B. Rutherford is in violation of the Standards by failing to deal with clients fairly in disseminating material changes in investment recommendations.
    C. Saris Corporation is in violation of the Standards by not disclosing material earnings information to the public.

12. Carlos Mendez, CFA, is beginning an investment advisory relationship with a new client and plans to formulate an investment policy statement (IPS) for the client. According to the Standard concerning suitability, Mendez is *least likely* to consider the client's:
    A. regulatory and legal circumstances.
    B. conflicts of interest.
    C. performance measurement benchmarks.

13. Chuck Hill, CFA, the financial manager of Niseron Corp., has just learned that Niseron's quarterly net income will fall well short of consensus analyst expectations. Hill decides that he should immediately notify analysts covering Niseron of this negative development. He calls two particular analysts first who have followed Niseron stock for several years and have alerted Hill to important developments at competing firms. Failing to notify these analysts might damage Hill's ability to monitor his competition, to the detriment of his own shareholders. Under CFA Institute's Code and Standards, Hill should *most* appropriately:
    A. notify no analysts until he is ready to issue the final numbers for the quarter.
    B. notify the two analysts first because their information adds value for Niseron's shareholders.
    C. issue a press release regarding Niseron's earnings prior to calling analysts.

14. Jim Gordon, CFA, is long 20,000 shares of ABC stock. The stock has recently declined below his original cost and Gordon would like to utilize the loss in calculating his income taxes for the current year. Gordon believes the stock will recover quickly, but he must sell the stock to realize the loss. Repurchasing the stock immediately would be considered a wash sale under income tax law and would negate the recognition of the loss. Gordon decides to sell ABC and use derivative instruments to create a synthetic long position.

    George Turpin, a CFA Level I candidate, has decided to enter into a sizeable long position of DEF stock. Since DEF is thinly traded, Turpin is concerned the order will overwhelm the liquidity of DEF and the price will surge. Turpin engages in a series of block trades to accomplish the purchase.

    According to CFA Institute Standards of Professional Conduct:
    A. Gordon is in violation of the Standards, but Turpin is not in violation.
    B. both Gordon and Turpin are in violation of the Standards.
    C. neither Gordon nor Turpin is in violation of the Standards.

15. Jenny Pickler, a Level II CFA Candidate, writes an economic forecast containing several interest rate projections. Her firm's investment committee reviews Pickler's report and changes several of the interest rates Pickler had forecast. To comply with CFA Institute Standards, Pickler:
    A. does not need to take any further action.
    B. should ask that her name be removed from the report.
    C. must independently review the data supporting the investment committee's changes.

16. John Malone, CFA, manages pension funds at BNA Trust Company. Malone's wife is on the board of directors of Barley Corporation and owns 3% of its outstanding stock. BNA Trust's research division has recently recommended Barley stock to its trust officers and pension fund portfolio managers. Based on the CFA Institute Standards, Malone:
    A. may purchase the stock after disclosing his spouse's ownership interest to his supervisor and to the trustees of the pension funds he manages.
    B. may not purchase the stock because he is not able to be unbiased and objective, given his spouse's affiliation with Barley.
    C. is free to act with no restrictions because he is not a beneficial owner of the Barley stock.

17. Denise Chavez, CFA, is the senior energy analyst for a major brokerage firm. Chavez is also a social and environmental activist, and is opposed to coal-fired power plants. She has been arrested twice for trespassing during organized pickets at some of these power plants. Chavez has recently accepted a volunteer position as Board member of Greensleeves, a foundation that lobbies governments on environmental issues. The position will involve significant volunteer hours, including some travel. Are Chavez's activities consistent with CFA Institute Standards?
    A. Chavez violated the Standards by being arrested, but the volunteer Board position is not a violation.
    B. The environmental activism is not a violation, but the Standards prohibit Chavez from accepting the Board position.
    C. The activism and subsequent arrests are not a violation, but Chavez must disclose the Board position to her employer.

18. Laura Smith, CFA, is an analyst with the trust department of Bright Star Bank. The department's portfolio managers use a proprietary model to select stocks. Bright Star has been purchased by Mega Bank, which does not plan to use Bright Star's model after completing the purchase. A few weeks before the Bright Star/Mega Bank merger date, Smith downloads the model to her laptop and modifies the model for her own use. Do Smith's actions violate the Standards of Professional Conduct?
    A. No, because Smith modified the model.
    B. Yes, because the model is the property of Mega Bank.
    C. No, because Mega Bank has discontinued use of the model.

Questions 19 through 32 relate to Quantitative Methods. (21 minutes)

19. George Reilly, CFA, manages the Ivy Foundation portfolio. The Ivy Foundation has a minimum acceptable return of 7%. The current risk-free rate is 6%. Reilly assumes that returns are normally distributed and wants to choose the optimal portfolio for the foundation. The *best* approach Reilly should take is to choose the portfolio that:
A. maximizes the Sharpe ratio.
B. maximizes the safety-first ratio.
C. minimizes the standard deviation of returns.

20. Returns data for Limbo Company exhibit the following statistics:
- Mean 9.5%
- Median 14.3%
- Excess Kurtosis –0.97

The returns distribution for Limbo Company is:
A. positively skewed.
B. negatively skewed.
C. not skewed.

21. Jack Smith, CFA, is the chief economist for Gable Investments. He believes that, in general, recessions result from increases in energy prices. Smith has estimated that in his home country the probability of a recession given higher oil prices is 40%. Smith also believes that there is a 30% probability oil prices will increase. The probability of observing rising oil prices and a recession is *closest* to:
A. 12%.
B. 18%.
C. 28%.

22. After repeatedly sampling the 1-year returns on the common stock of Bernouli Inc., a semiconductor manufacturer, an analyst notices that the returns conform to a normal probability distribution. Which of the following statements *correctly* describes the returns on Bernouli's common stock?
A. The mean value is greater than the median.
B. Large deviations from the mean are less likely than small deviations.
C. The distributions can be completely described by the residual value and the standard deviation.

23. Frank Jones is considering three separate investments. Investment 1 pays a stated annual interest rate of 6.1%, compounded annually. Investment 2 pays a stated annual interest rate of 6.0%, compounded monthly. Investment 3 pays a stated annual interest rate of 5.9%, compounded quarterly. Which investment should Smith choose?
A. Investment 1.
B. Investment 2.
C. Investment 3.

24. Sean Dahib, a quantitative analyst, has been given the assignment of tallying the P/Es of the companies in an index of 500 stocks. He constructs the following table:

P/Es	# of Companies
0 up to 10	25
10 up to 20	100
20 up to 30	150
30 up to 40	145
40 up to 50	35
50 up to 60	25
60 up to 70	10
70 up to 80	10

What is the relative class frequency for the class of companies with the smallest P/Es?
A. 12.5%.
B. 5.0%.
C. 2.0%.

25. Alice Morton, CFA, is reviewing a research paper that reaches a conclusion based on two hypothesis tests with *p*-values of 0.037 and 0.064. Morton should conclude that:
A. both of these tests' null hypotheses can be rejected with 90% confidence.
B. neither of these tests' null hypotheses can be rejected with 95% confidence.
C. only one of these tests' null hypotheses can be rejected with 99% confidence.

26. Lee Pickett, CFA, is forecasting next year's earnings for Stonewall Company using a probability model. Pickett believes the probability that Stonewall's earnings will increase in the next year depends on whether interest rates increase. Pickett constructs the following tree diagram:

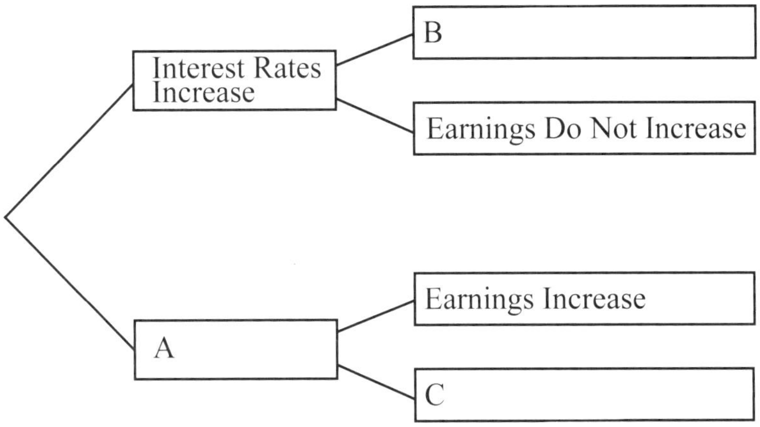

In this tree diagram:
A. Cell A represents the unconditional probability that interest rates do not increase.
B. Cell B represents the conditional probability that interest rates increase, given that earnings increase.
C. Cell C represents the conditional probability that earnings do not increase, given that interest rates increase.

27. If a one-tailed *z*-test uses a 5% significance level, the test will reject a:
A. true null hypothesis 5% of the time.
B. false null hypothesis 95% of the time.
C. true null hypothesis 95% of the time.

28. Burle Weaver and Jane Palmer, analysts for Growthmore Managers, are assigned the task of examining the mean return for growth stocks. After sorting 10,000 stocks based on price-to-earnings ratios, Weaver and Palmer classify the stocks with price-to earnings ratios above the median as growth stocks. They then use a random number generator to select a sample of 100 stocks from the growth stocks. In his meeting with the Growthmore board, Weaver states that his sampling procedure is an example of stratified random sampling. Palmer explains that the distribution of the 100 sampled stocks is called a sampling distribution. Determine whether the statements made by Weaver and Palmer are correct.
A. Only Weaver is incorrect.
B. Only Palmer is incorrect.
C. Both Weaver and Palmer are incorrect.

29. On a point-and-figure chart, each unit on the horizontal axis represents a(n):
A. equal time period.
B. specific number of shares traded.
C. change in direction of the price trend.

30. Jon Pelker plans to retire in six years and will require $950,000. Today, Pelker will deposit $100,000 into an interest bearing account and will deposit an additional $100,000 at the end of each of the next six years. What annual percentage return must Pelker earn to achieve his goal of $950,000 for his retirement?
A. 8%.
B. 10%.
C. 18%.

31. Gus Hayden is evaluating the performance of the portfolio manager in charge of his retirement account. The account started with $5,000,000 and generated a 15% return in year 1 and a –5% return in year 2. Hayden adds $2,000,000 at the beginning of year 2. Hayden added $2,000,000 to the account at the beginning of year 2. The appropriately measured annualized return is *closest* to:
A. 3.0%.
B. 4.5%.
C. 9.0%.

32. Kidra Rao ranks and classifies firms into ten groups based on their interest coverage ratios, lowest to highest. Rao's ranking system is *best* described as a(n):
A. ratio scale.
B. nominal scale.
C. ordinal scale.

Questions 33 through 44 relate to Economics. (18 minutes)

33. The short run, as an economic decision-making time frame, is *best* described as:
A. one year or the length of the firm's production cycle.
B. the period during which the firm's plant size and production methods are fixed.
C. the period in which the firm cannot change its input quantities of labor and materials.

34. The market supply and demand curves for a good are $P = 0.05Q_S + 0.84$ and $P = 180 - 0.25Q_D$. At a market price of 30, the market excess demand is *closest* to:
A. 9 units.
B. 17 units.
C. 32 units.

35. In the chain of events by which monetary policy affects the economy, which is *most likely* to have limitations that make a policy action less effective in achieving its desired outcome?
A. Changes in interbank lending rates are reflected in other short-term interest rates.
B. Long-term interest rates change in response to changes in short-term interest rates.
C. Central bank purchases or sales of securities change the amount of excess reserves in the banking system.

36. The U.S. Federal Reserve is *most likely* to purchase Treasury securities in the open market when:
A. it believes interest rates are too low to achieve its primary goal of price level stability.
B. it believes lower interest rates will reduce the M1 measure to its intermediate target level.
C. the federal funds rate is higher than the Fed's target rate.

37. The consumer price index is *best* described as:
A. the inflation rate for a given period of time.
B. an unbiased estimate of changes in the cost of living.
C. a weighted average cost for a basket of goods and services.

38. As a result of a decline in cucumber production by small-scale growers, the U.S. government has decided to provide assistance to cucumber growers by paying them $0.05 per pound produced. Which of the following is the *most likely* result of this policy?
A. The marginal benefit of cucumbers will exceed the marginal cost, causing a deadweight loss.
B. The marginal cost of cucumbers will exceed the marginal benefit, causing a deadweight loss.
C. The marginal cost of cucumbers will exceed the marginal benefit, and a shortage of cucumbers will emerge.

39. Based on the aggregate demand/aggregate supply model:
A. an inflationary or recessionary gap may exist in the long run.
B. actual real GDP is equal to potential real GDP in the long run.
C. no upward or downward pressure on the price level is present at short-run equilibrium.

40. Assume the exchange rate between the Bucas (BCS) and the Leider (LDR) is 1.70 BCS/LDR, and the exchange rate between the Bucas and the Passoa (PAS) is 3.2 BCS/PAS. The PAS/LDR exchange rate is *closest* to:
A. 0.5313 PAS/LDR.
B. 1.8824 PAS/LDR.
C. 5.4400 PAS/LDR.

41. Tetra Corporation holds the exclusive production rights to a wireless cellular phone technology. Tetra's production rights will remain exclusive for 15 years, effectively eliminating any competition while the technology is viable. If their marginal revenue, marginal cost, and average total cost are $50, $43, and $57, respectively, Tetra Corporation can maximize profits by:
A. expanding output until marginal revenue equals marginal cost.
B. reducing output until marginal revenue equals average total cost.
C. expanding output until marginal revenue equals average total cost.

42. Wilmer Jones owns several restaurants in different cities. His restaurants compete on quality of food and service, price, and marketing. Competitors can enter and exit his markets, and there are usually several competitors in each market. His market structure can *best* be characterized as:
A. perfect competition.
B. monopolistic competition.
C. oligopoly.

43. The country of Colfax uses 10 units of labor to produce a unit of rice and 15 units of labor to produce a unit of plastic. The country of Birklund uses 12 units of labor to produce a unit of rice and 18 units of labor to produce a unit of plastic. With regard to potential benefits of trading rice and plastic between Colfax and Birklund:
A. there are no potential gains from trade.
B. Colfax should produce and trade rice for Birklund's plastic.
C. Birklund should produce and trade rice for Colfax's plastic.

44. In measures of national economic output, realized capital gains on assets purchased in an earlier period are a component of:
A. gross domestic product, but not gross national product.
B. gross national product, but not gross domestic product.
C. neither gross domestic product nor gross national product.

Questions 45 through 68 relate to Financial Reporting and Analysis. (36 minutes)

45. Information about any conflicts of interest between management, the board of directors, and shareholders can *most likely* be found in the:
A. proxy statement.
B. footnotes.
C. auditor's report.

46. Which one of the following accounts *least likely* describes a current asset?
A. Trade receivables.
B. Prepaid expenses.
C. Strategic investments.

47. Degen, Inc., owns a trademark which it originally valued at €15 million on its balance sheet but currently values at €10 million. In the country where Degen is incorporated, trademarks are protected by law for as long as their owner remains a going concern. Degen has *most likely*:
    A. developed its trademark at a cost of €15 million.
    B. recorded amortization expense of €5 million on its trademark.
    C. recognized €5 million of impairment charges on its trademark.

48. A profitable company can increase its return on equity (other things equal) by:
    A. decreasing its asset turnover.
    B. increasing its financial leverage.
    C. decreasing its ratio of EBT to EBIT.

49. GreenCo, a U.S.-based manufacturing firm, reports a deferred tax liability on its balance sheet. The deferred tax liability *most likely* results from GreenCo's:
    A. use of the last-in-first-out inventory accounting method for its financial statements.
    B. use of straight line depreciation for financial reporting and accelerated depreciation for tax purposes.
    C. decision to expense restructuring costs on its income statement even though the funds have not been paid.

50. A company reports the following unusual events:
    - Loss on discontinued operations.
    - Restructuring and severance costs applicable to asset sales.
    - Plant shutdown costs.

    Which of these items would *most likely* be considered nonrecurring and included in operating income?
    A. Restructuring and severance costs applicable to asset sales and plant shutdown costs.
    B. Loss on discontinued operations and restructuring and severance costs applicable to asset sales.
    C. Loss on discontinued operations and plant shutdown costs.

51. Deferred tax assets result from:
    A. gains that are recognized in the income statement before they are taxable, while deferred tax liabilities result from gains that are taxable before they are recognized in the income statement.
    B. gains that are taxable before they are recognized in the income statement, while deferred tax liabilities result from gains that are recognized in the income statement before they are taxable.
    C. losses that are tax deductible before they are recognized in the income statement, while deferred tax liabilities result from losses that are recognized in the income statement before they are tax deductible.

52. At the beginning of the year, Weatherford Corporation had 2,000,000 shares of common stock outstanding. In addition, Weatherford had 150,000 stock options outstanding to purchase common shares at $10 per share. No stock options were exercised during the year. Assuming the average market price of the stock was $15, how many shares should Weatherford use in computing diluted earnings per share for the year?
    A. 2,000,000.
    B. 2,050,000.
    C. 2,150,000.

53. Fasimath Company's earnings before interest and taxes (EBIT) and interest coverage ratio for the most recent year are unchanged from the prior year, but its fixed charge coverage ratio has decreased. This *most likely* suggests that Fasimath's:
    A. working capital has decreased.
    B. lease payments have increased.
    C. financial leverage has increased.

54. Jansen Co., a manufacturer of high-end sports equipment, earned $45 million in net income for the year. The company paid out $1.30 per share in dividends. Jansen issued 500,000 shares at the beginning of the year at $20 (1 million shares were outstanding before the issuance). The market value of Jansen's trading securities decreased by $2.4 million. The increase in Jansen's stockholders' equity is *closest* to:
    A. $43 million.
    B. $51 million.
    C. $53 million.

55. Soft Inc., which follows U.S. GAAP, sells $100 million of common stock, pays $15 million in interest, records $23 million of depreciation, acquires a software company for $175 million, sells a product line for $86 million, pays $13 million in dividends, and contributes $50 million to a joint venture. Cash flow from investing (CFI) for Soft is:
A. –$139 million.
B. –$152 million.
C. –$167 million.

56. Joplin Corporation reports the following in its year-end financial statements:
- Net income of $43.7 million.
- Depreciation expense of $4.2 million.
- Increase in accounts receivable of $1.5 million.
- Decrease in accounts payable of $2.3 million.
- Increase in capital stock of $50 million.
- Sold equipment with a book value of $7 million for $15 million after-tax.
- Purchased equipment for $35 million.

Joplin's free cash flow to the firm (FCFF) is *closest* to:
A. $16 million.
B. $24 million.
C. $66 million.

57. Stanley Electronics reports the following information:

Beginning inventory	100 units	$15
Purchases	200 units	$21
	100 units	$18
	300 units	$24
Ending inventory	150 units	

Cost of goods sold (COGS) for a periodic inventory system using the average cost inventory method is *closest* to:
A. $11,100.
B. $11,550.
C. $12,150.

58. Ecker Company has both a deferred tax asset and a deferred tax liability on its balance sheet that were created when its statutory tax rate was 30%. If Ecker's tax rate increases to 35%, the value of Ecker's deferred tax items will:

	Deferred tax asset	Deferred tax liability
A.	Increase	Decrease
B.	Decrease	Increase
C.	Increase	Increase

59. Which of the following statements *most accurately* describes the general features of financial statements under IFRS?
    A. Each of the required financial statements is prepared using accrual accounting.
    B. Assets may not be offset against liabilities unless specifically permitted or required by a standard.
    C. Prior-period information may only be presented when specifically permitted or required by a standard.

60. Investing cash flows *most likely* reflect changes in which of the firm's balance sheet items?
    A. Noncurrent assets.
    B. Noncurrent liabilities and equity.
    C. Current assets and current liabilities.

61. Three years ago, Jegich Company acquired an asset to be used in manufacturing its products. Recently, Jegich determined that the future undiscounted cash flows associated with the asset exceed the asset's carrying value. In addition, it is determined that the carrying value of the asset exceeds its fair value. According to U.S. GAAP, with the asset at its current carrying value, Jegich's return on equity:
    A. is overstated, and the total asset turnover is understated.
    B. and total asset turnover are both overstated.
    C. and total asset turnover are both correctly stated.

62. Upton Corporation has the following capital structure:

Upton Capital Structure	*Shares*
Cumulative Preferred Stock \$100 par value pays \$6.50 per share	20,000
Common stock	500,000

Upton's 20X8 net income was \$830,000 and the company's tax rate was 35%.

The 20X8 basic earnings per share for Upton Corporation is *closest* to:
    A. \$1.40.
    B. \$1.60.
    C. \$1.66.

63. XYZ Company has decided to issue $10 million of unsecured bonds. If issued today, the 4% semi-annual coupon bonds would require a market interest rate of 12%. Under U.S. GAAP, how will these bonds affect XYZ's statement of cash flows?
   A. The coupon payments will decrease operating cash flow each year and the discount will decrease financing cash flow at maturity.
   B. The periodic interest expense will decrease operating cash flow and the discount will decrease financing cash flow at maturity.
   C. The coupon payments and the discount amortization will decrease financing cash flow each year.

64. Attitudes and rationalizations that may lead to accounting fraud *most likely* include:
   A. ineffective monitoring by management.
   B. risks to the personal wealth of company managers.
   C. commitments to outside parties to meet aggressive goals.

65. Sanders Company recently leased equipment used in its manufacturing operation. For financial reporting purposes, Sanders treated the transaction as an operating lease. George Batter, CFA, believes that Sanders should have capitalized the lease, and he adjusts Sanders' financial statement to reflect his view. Batter's adjustments will *most likely*:
   A. decrease Sanders' debt-to-capital ratio.
   B. increase Sanders' return on equity in the early years of the lease and decrease it in the later years.
   C. decrease Sanders' interest coverage ratio.

66. Mullins Company's financial statements include an auditor's report with a qualified opinion. This *most likely* implies that the:
   A. auditor is reasonably assured that the financial statements are free of material errors.
   B. financial statements include exceptions to the applicable accounting standards but are presented fairly.
   C. financial statements are materially out of compliance with the applicable accounting standards and are not presented fairly.

67. A company purchases an asset in the first quarter and decides to capitalize the asset. Compared to expensing the asset cost, capitalizing the asset cost will result in higher cash flows in the first quarter from:
   A. investing.
   B. financing.
   C. operations.

68. Under U.S. GAAP, the completed contract method of revenue recognition for a long-term project:
A. is appropriate when the project's costs or revenues cannot be estimated reliably.
B. specifies that the profit or loss from the project is recognized only when the project is completed.
C. permits profit from the project to be recognized during construction to the extent that cash collected is greater than costs incurred.

Questions 69 through 78 relate to Corporate Finance. (15 minutes)

69. ChemCo is evaluating a project based on the principles of capital budgeting. ChemCo should accept the project if it has a:
A. net present value equal to zero.
B. profitability index greater than one.
C. required rate of return greater than its internal rate of return.

70. Mentemeyer Corporation is a small firm that needs to increase short-term liquidity but has weak credit. The source of short-term financing that would *most likely* be available to Mentemeyer is:
A. commercial paper.
B. nonbank finance companies.
C. a revolving credit agreement.

71. Two of the typical steps in the capital budgeting process are:
A. analyzing project proposals and raising additional capital.
B. raising additional capital and creating the firm-wide capital budget.
C. analyzing project proposals and creating the firm-wide capital budget.

72. The asset beta of a firm equals its equity beta if:
A. the company has no debt.
B. the company has no equity.
C. the company's debt equals its equity.

73. Over the next year, Thatherton Co. is expecting their marginal tax rate to increase by 5%. Also, over the next 12 months, Thatherton plans to undertake several expansion projects significantly more risky than previous projects. Thatherton Co.'s current capital structure includes 40% debt and 60% equity. Which of the following statements *correctly* summarizes the effect these changes will have on the company's marginal cost of capital?
A. The increasing tax rate will increase the MCC.
B. The riskier projects will increase the MCC.
C. Both the increasing tax rate and the riskier projects will increase the MCC.

74. The interests of shareowners are *most likely* to be protected by a board member election policy that:
A. allows shareowners to remove a board member.
B. staggers the multiple-year terms of board members.
C. allows the board to fill a vacant position for the remainder of a term.

75. Nagle Company produces a commodity with a market price of $3.25 per unit. Nagle forecasts production and sales of 900,000 units over the next quarter. Nagle's variable cost per unit is $3.75, and fixed operating costs are $400,000. Based on these projections, it is *most likely* that:
A. Nagle's contribution margin for the quarter is $0.50 per unit.
B. Nagle will experience an operating loss of $400,000 for the quarter.
C. Nagle's breakeven quantity of sales for the quarter is 1,200,000 units.

76. An analyst has discovered that over the last three years, Gathers Company has experienced a decrease in its net operating cycle, while over the same time period the average net operating cycle for the industry (excluding Gathers) has increased. These trends *most likely* indicate that:
A. Gathers has decreased its liquidity position by increasing the amount of time inventory spends in its warehouses.
B. Gathers has increased its liquidity position by increasing the speed of cash collection from its customers.
C. the industry has decreased its liquidity position by increasing the average amount of time to pay suppliers.

77. An analyst is reviewing the working capital portfolio investment policy of a publicly traded firm. Which of the following components of the policy is the analyst *least likely* to find acceptable?
A. Investments must have an A-1 rating from S&P or an equivalent rating from another agency.
B. Authority for selecting and managing short-term investments rests with the firm's treasurer and any designees selected by the treasurer.
C. Investments in U.S. T-bills, commercial paper, and bank CDs are acceptable unless issued by Stratford Bank.

78. The audit committee for a firm is *most likely* to represent shareowners' interests if:
A. the external auditor submits its auditing reports to the firm's chief financial officer.
B. the majority of the audit committee members also hold positions within the firm.
C. shareowners vote to approve external auditors nominated by the audit committee.

Questions 79 through 84 relate to Portfolio Management. (9 minutes)

79. Bruce Johansen, CFA, is fully invested in the market portfolio. Johansen desires to increase the expected return from his portfolio. According to capital market theory, Johansen can meet his return objective *best* by:
 A. allocating a higher proportion of the portfolio to higher risk assets.
 B. borrowing at the risk-free rate to invest in the risky market portfolio.
 C. owning the risky market portfolio and lending at the risk-free rate.

80. Beta of an asset is calculated as the covariance of the asset's returns with market returns:
 A. divided by the variance of market returns.
 B. divided by the standard deviation of the asset's returns.
 C. multiplied by the ratio of the asset's standard deviation of returns to the market's standard deviation of returns.

81. A risk averse investor is *best* described as an individual who:
 A. only invests in risk-free investments.
 B. will choose a relatively low-risk portfolio.
 C. prefers investments with less risk to those with more risk if they have the same expected return.

82. The standard deviation of a two-stock portfolio *least likely:*
 A. is less than or equal to the weighted average of the two assets' standard deviations.
 B. can be reduced by increasing the relative weight of the stock with a lower standard deviation.
 C. will be minimized when the correlation between the two stocks equals zero.

83. An analyst predicts that the return on Royal Company stock will be 15%. The analyst is provided with the following data for Royal and the broad market:
 - Royal Company beta 1.5
 - Risk-free rate 5%
 - Expected market return 11%

 Based on these data, the analyst should conclude that Royal Company stock is:
 A. overvalued.
 B. undervalued.
 C. correctly valued.

84. Marcia Kostner, CFA, is an advisor to individual investors. To determine each of her clients' risk tolerance objectively, Kostner uses a mathematical formula with inputs that include the client's age, family size, insurance coverage, liquidity, income, and net worth. What is the *most likely* shortcoming of Kostner's approach to assessing risk tolerance?
A. Net worth is unrelated to an investor's risk tolerance.
B. This approach does not consider the investor's attitude toward risk.
C. Treating clients differently based on their ages violates the Code and Standards.

Questions 85 through 96 relate to Equity Investments. (18 minutes)

85. Malley, Inc., is a manufacturer of sports apparel. Pruett, Inc., produces cardboard boxes for packaging. In a typical industry classification system from a commercial index provider, in which sectors are these firms *most likely* to be classified?

	<u>Malley, Inc.</u>	<u>Pruett, Inc.</u>
A.	Consumer staples	Basic materials and processing
B.	Consumer discretionary	Basic materials and processing
C.	Consumer staples	Industrial and producer durables

86. Assuming the value effect persists over time, which of the following strategies would be *most likely* to earn positive abnormal returns? Purchase stocks with:
A. low dividend yields.
B. high market-to-book ratios.
C. low price-to-earnings ratios.

87. Roger Gould, CFA, is analyzing the stock of Zero Incorporated and trying to determine which price multiple to use in his valuation. Zero, a start-up, had losses over the last 12 months and is projected to have a loss over the next 12 months. Zero has significant internally generated intangible assets and human capital that Gould would like to capture in his valuation. The price multiple that Gould should *most* appropriately use is the:
A. price-to-sales ratio.
B. price-to-book value.
C. price-to-earnings ratio.

88. In the industry life cycle model, the threat of new entrants into an industry is greatest during the:
A. mature stage.
B. growth stage.
C. embryonic stage.

89. Participating preference shares are *most* accurately described as preferred stock that:
A. may be exchanged for the firm's common shares at a predetermined ratio.
B. receives extra dividends if the firm's profits are greater than a predetermined level.
C. must be paid any omitted dividends from prior periods before the firm may pay dividends to common shareholders.

90. Agriff Company paid a dividend of $1.90 per share last year. Dividends are expected to grow at a constant rate of 6%. The risk-free rate is 5%, the market risk premium is 7%, and the beta of the common shares is 1.3. The value of the Agriff Company's common shares is *closest* to:
A. $23.46.
B. $24.86.
C. $33.57.

91. Which of the following types of index is *least likely* to require frequent reconstitution of constituent securities?
A. Equity index.
B. Commodity index.
C. Fixed income index.

92. The derivative pricing rule on an electronic crossing network states that orders will execute at a price determined by:
A. the price of the security's underlying asset.
B. quotes on the exchange where the asset is listed.
C. matching the buy and sell orders on the crossing network.

93. Willa Dowd collected the following information for a small-cap firm that she is evaluating:

• Stock price per share	$20.50
• Expected sales	$920 million
• Operating expenses (excluding interest)	$405 million
• Depreciation & amortization	$44 million
• Return on equity (ROE)	12%
• Shares outstanding	31 million
• Common shareholders' equity	$380 million

The price/cash flow ratio for the small-cap firm is *closest* to:
A. 7.1.
B. 8.5.
C. 9.1.

94. Kate Johnson, CFA, owns shares of a stock that currently trades at $15. If Johnson wants to buy more shares if the price increases to $17, she should enter a:
A. stop buy order at $17.
B. limit order to buy at $17.
C. market order to buy at $17.

95. James Fry, CFA, is evaluating the potential investment merit of Cushing Corporation. Cushing's most recent year's earnings were $5.00 per share, and Cushing paid a dividend of $1.50 per share. Fry forecasts that Cushing will earn $4.70 per share next year. Fry estimates Cushing's future growth rate will be 10%, with a required rate of return of 12%. Based on the information provided, Cushing's leading price to earnings (P/E) ratio is *closest* to:
A. 15.0.
B. 15.9.
C. 17.6.

96. A 5.8% preferred stock with a par value of $1,000 has an annual yield of 5.4%. A zero-coupon bond with a face value of $1,000 will mature in 3 years and has a yield of 4.7%. Which security has a higher price today?
A. The preferred stock.
B. The zero-coupon bond.
C. Their prices today are equal.

Questions 97 through 110 relate to Fixed Income. (21 minutes)

97. An analyst has stated that, holding all else constant, an increase in the maturity of a coupon bond will increase its interest rate risk, and that a decrease in the coupon rate of a coupon bond will decrease its interest rate risk. The analyst is correct with respect to:
A. both of these effects.
B. neither of these effects.
C. only one of these effects.

98. Which of the following embedded bond options tends to benefit the borrower?
A. Put option.
B. Interest rate cap.
C. Conversion option.

99. Chris South owns $25,000 face value of Bradco bonds, which have a 7% coupon, pay interest semiannually, and have six years remaining until maturity. The bonds are callable at par. The bonds were rated A when Chris bought them at par two years ago, and they are currently worth $26,225, with a rating of AA. Over this 2-year period, the Bradco bonds have experienced a(n):
A. decrease in call risk.
B. increase in liquidity risk.
C. decrease in credit risk.

100. The government of the Holmen Islands has one issue of bonds outstanding, with an annual coupon of 6% and a maturity date of September 2027. One year after these bonds were issued, their yield to maturity has decreased to 5%, and the government uses a tap system to issue new bonds. The newly issued bonds are *most likely*:
A. 5% coupon bonds maturing in September 2028.
B. 6% coupon bonds maturing in September 2027.
C. 6% coupon bonds maturing in September 2028.

101. If a callable bond has an option-adjusted spread (OAS) of 75 basis points, this *most likely* suggests:
A. the bond has a zero-volatility spread greater than 75 basis points.
B. the implied cost of the call option is the bond's nominal spread minus 75 basis points.
C. the 75 basis points represent the investor's compensation for credit risk, liquidity risk, and volatility risk.

102. Bond X is a noncallable corporate bond maturing in ten years. Bond Y is also a corporate bond maturing in ten years, but Bond Y is callable at any time beginning three years from now. Both bonds carry a credit rating of AA. Based on this information:
A. Bond Y will have a higher nominal spread over a 10-year U.S. Treasury security than Bond X.
B. The option adjusted spread of Bond Y will be greater than its nominal spread.
C. The nominal spread of Bond X will be greater than its option adjusted spread.

103. A Treasury bond dealer observes the following Treasury spot rates, expressed as bond-equivalent yields: 6-month 7.4%, 12-month 7.0%, and 18-month 6.3%. The dealer also observes that the market price of an 8% coupon Treasury note with 18 months to maturity is $1,019.50. The dealer can earn:
A. no arbitrage profit because the 8% coupon bond is selling for its arbitrage-free price.
B. an arbitrage profit by buying the 8% coupon bond in the open market, stripping it, and selling the pieces.
C. an arbitrage profit by selling the 8% coupon bond short and buying the component cash flow STRIPs with the proceeds.

104. David Garcia, CFA, is analyzing two bonds. Bond X is an option-free coupon bond with ten years to maturity. Bond Y is a mortgage-backed security that also matures in ten years. Garcia is considering two possible interest rate scenarios—one in which rates are flat over the entire 10-year horizon, and one in which the yield curve is sloped steeply upward. For each bond, Garcia calculates the nominal spread over the 10-year U.S. Treasury issue as well as the zero-volatility spread. The zero-volatility spread is *most* different from the nominal spread:
A. for Bond X and an upward sloping yield curve.
B. for Bond Y and an upward sloping yield curve.
C. for Bond Y and a flat yield curve.

105. Which of the following bonds is *least likely* to exhibit negative convexity?
A. Putable bond.
B. Callable bond.
C. Mortgage passthrough.

106. When calculating and interpreting a firm's leverage and coverage ratios, which component of traditional credit analysis is an analyst *most likely* addressing?
A. Capacity.
B. Character.
C. Collateral.

107. Kathy Hurst, CFA, is valuing a 4-year zero coupon security and has acquired the following information:

1-year spot rate	6.0%
4-year spot rate	7.5%
1-year forward rate 1 year from now	7.3%
1-year forward rate 3 years from now	8.9%

The 1-year forward rate 2 years from now is *closest* to:
A. 7.3%.
B. 7.8%.
C. 8.0%.

108. ABC Corporation has just issued $200 million of 6.5% $1,000 par value bonds at face value. Which of the following requirements in the indenture for these bonds would *most likely* be considered a negative covenant? ABC must:
A. maintain its manufacturing equipment in good condition.
B. make timely semiannual payments of interest and principal when due.
C. have paid all bond coupon payments due before it can pay cash dividends.

109. Original maturities on U.S. Treasury notes:
A. are less than 1 year.
B. range from 2 to 10 years.
C. range up to 30 years.

110. Inflation risk in bond investing is *best* described as the risk that the:
A. value of a bond's payments will decline in terms of real goods and services.
B. realized yield will be less than the bond's yield to maturity as of the purchase date.
C. price of a bond will respond more to an increase in interest rates than to an equal-sized decrease in interest rates.

Questions 111 through 116 relate to Derivatives. (9 minutes)

111. Roland Carlson owns a portfolio of large capitalization stocks. Carlson has a positive long-term outlook for the stock market, but would like to protect his portfolio from any sudden declines in the stock market, without selling his holdings. The *most likely* way for Carlson to achieve his objective of limiting the downside risk of his portfolio is to:
A. sell put options on the S&P 500.
B. sell an S&P 500 futures contract.
C. buy an S&P 500 forward contract.

112. Julia Chen, a portfolio manager for U.S.-based Dane Investments, establishes a short position in Swiss franc currency futures. The position consists of 100,000 contracts with an initial margin of $4,000, a maintenance margin of $2,500, and a contract price of 0.9120 USD/CHF. If the futures price on the subsequent two days is 0.9300 and 0.8928, respectively, Chen's margin account balance at the end of the second day is *closest* to:
A. $4,000.
B. $5,920.
C. $7,720.

113. The underlying rate for a LIBOR-based 3 × 6 forward rate agreement is:
A. 60-day LIBOR.
B. 90-day LIBOR.
C. 180-day LIBOR.

114. Call options on the stock of Verdant, Inc., with a strike price of $45 are priced at $3.75. Put options with a strike price of $45 are priced at $3.00. If the writers and buyers of these options do not have underlying positions in Verdant stock:
A. the call writer has more loss exposure than the put buyer.
B. the put buyer has more loss exposure than the put writer.
C. the put writer has a larger potential gain than the call buyer.

115. An option that gives the owner the right to sell 100 shares of stock only on the expiration date three months from now at a strike price of $35, when the current stock price is $25, is an:
A. out-of-the-money American put option.
B. in-the-money European put option.
C. out-of-the-money European put option.

116. Irczek Investments is actively engaged in various risk management strategies involving swaps. The company currently has a position as the fixed rate payer in a quarterly fixed-for-equity swap with an interest rate of 8%, a tenor of five years and notional principal of $10 million. Payments on the swap are netted. The underlying equity return is based on the S&P 500 Index. Irczek currently owes a payment of $400,000. The underlying equity index:
A. decreased by 2% in the last quarter.
B. was unchanged in the last quarter.
C. increased by 2% in the last quarter.

Questions 117 through 120 relate to Alternative Investments. (6 minutes)

117. With respect to mezzanine-stage financing in venture capital investing and mezzanine financing of a leveraged buyout:
    A. mezzanine-stage financing refers to a type of security but mezzanine financing does not.
    B. mezzanine financing refers to a type of security but mezzanine-stage financing does not.
    C. both terms refer financing by issuance of securities that have both debt and equity characteristics.

118. An investor in a hedge fund that holds some thinly traded securities is wondering about how the net asset value is calculated for the hedge fund's financial statements. He should know that on the financial statements, net asset values are *most likel*y calculated using the:
    A. average of the bid and ask for traded securities.
    B. bid for short positions and the ask for long positions.
    C. average quote for traded securities less a liquidity discount.

119. Because of survivorship bias, hedge fund data are *most likely* to:
    A. overstate returns and overstate risk.
    B. overstate returns and understate risk.
    C. understate returns and overstate risk.

120. A commodity market is in contango if the spot price is:
    A. higher than futures prices.
    B. equal to futures prices.
    C. lower than futures prices.

End of Afternoon Session

Exam 3
Morning Session

Topic	Questions	Points
Ethical and Professional Standards	1–18	27
Quantitative Methods	19–32	21
Economics	33–44	18
Financial Reporting and Analysis	45–68	36
Corporate Finance	69–78	15
Portfolio Management	79–84	9
Equity Investments	85–96	18
Fixed Income	97–110	21
Derivatives	111–116	9
Alternative Investments	117–120	6
Total		**180**

Test Answers

1.	A	B	C
2.	A	B	C
3.	A	B	C
4.	A	B	C
5.	A	B	C
6.	A	B	C
7.	A	B	C
8.	A	B	C
9.	A	B	C
10.	A	B	C
11.	A	B	C
12.	A	B	C
13.	A	B	C
14.	A	B	C
15.	A	B	C
16.	A	B	C
17.	A	B	C
18.	A	B	C
19.	A	B	C
20.	A	B	C
21.	A	B	C
22.	A	B	C
23.	A	B	C
24.	A	B	C
25.	A	B	C
26.	A	B	C
27.	A	B	C
28.	A	B	C
29.	A	B	C
30.	A	B	C
31.	A	B	C
32.	A	B	C
33.	A	B	C
34.	A	B	C
35.	A	B	C
36.	A	B	C
37.	A	B	C
38.	A	B	C
39.	A	B	C
40.	A	B	C
41.	A	B	C
42.	A	B	C
43.	A	B	C
44.	A	B	C
45.	A	B	C
46.	A	B	C
47.	A	B	C
48.	A	B	C
49.	A	B	C
50.	A	B	C
51.	A	B	C
52.	A	B	C
53.	A	B	C
54.	A	B	C
55.	A	B	C
56.	A	B	C
57.	A	B	C
58.	A	B	C
59.	A	B	C
60.	A	B	C
61.	A	B	C
62.	A	B	C
63.	A	B	C
64.	A	B	C
65.	A	B	C
66.	A	B	C
67.	A	B	C
68.	A	B	C
69.	A	B	C
70.	A	B	C
71.	A	B	C
72.	A	B	C
73.	A	B	C
74.	A	B	C
75.	A	B	C
76.	A	B	C
77.	A	B	C
78.	A	B	C
79.	A	B	C
80.	A	B	C
81.	A	B	C
82.	A	B	C
83.	A	B	C
84.	A	B	C
85.	A	B	C
86.	A	B	C
87.	A	B	C
88.	A	B	C
89.	A	B	C
90.	A	B	C
91.	A	B	C
92.	A	B	C
93.	A	B	C
94.	A	B	C
95.	A	B	C
96.	A	B	C
97.	A	B	C
98.	A	B	C
99.	A	B	C
100.	A	B	C
101.	A	B	C
102.	A	B	C
103.	A	B	C
104.	A	B	C
105.	A	B	C
106.	A	B	C
107.	A	B	C
108.	A	B	C
109.	A	B	C
110.	A	B	C
111.	A	B	C
112.	A	B	C
113.	A	B	C
114.	A	B	C
115.	A	B	C
116.	A	B	C
117.	A	B	C
118.	A	B	C
119.	A	B	C
120.	A	B	C

Exam 3
Morning Session

Questions 1 through 18 relate to Ethical and Professional Standards. (27 minutes)

1. Ryan Brown, CFA, is a portfolio manager for Brinton Investments. Brown has just issued a press release for Brinton regarding the CFA exam results for several of the company's analysts. The press release states the following: "Two of our analysts passed the Level III CFA exam this year after passing the prior two levels on the first attempt. These analysts have demonstrated Brinton's continued commitment to the highest standard of knowledge and ethics in the investment profession and will hopefully allow Brinton to continue its record of outstanding investment performance. Additionally, three other analysts passed the Level II CFA exam. These analysts will be able to identify themselves as CFA charterholders next year, a significant addition to the ten CFA charterholders already on staff." Did Brown violate the CFA Institute Standards of Professional Conduct with respect to his comments regarding Brinton's Level III or Level II CFA candidates?
   A. Both statements violate the Standards.
   B. Neither statement violates the Standards.
   C. Only one of the statements violates the Standards.

2. Julian Bates, CFA, is a research analyst who follows the airline industry. Bates has been asked to accompany two of his firm's salespeople to visit clients who have large holdings in the airline industry. Bates reviews reports by analysts from rival firms and discovers that another analyst has identified an issue that may hurt the airline industry over the next six months. Bates believes the other analyst's opinion is sound. At the first client meeting, Bates delivers his prepared presentation, and at the end, informs the client of "his important new discovery." According to the CFA Institute Standards of Professional Conduct, Bates has:
   A. not violated any Standard because his own research supports his conclusion.
   B. violated the Standards by misrepresenting the other analyst's idea as his own.
   C. violated the Standards by relying on research prepared by a competing firm.

3. Wendy Johnson, CFA, has recently been hired as a portfolio manager for Smith Brothers, an investment firm that caters to institutional clients. For the past five years, Johnson has provided investment advice to a local university. Johnson spends approximately five hours per week on the project. Johnson does not disclose this arrangement to her supervisor at Smith Brothers because the time involved will in no way interfere with her duties in her new position. Johnson has *most likely*:
   A. violated the Standards by failing to disclose a conflict of interest to her employer.
   B. violated the Standards by not obtaining permission from her employer.
   C. not violated any Standards.

4. Mark Hanning, CFA, is writing a research report on a firm. Hanning's supervisor, Rob Jannsen, sees a draft which includes favorable earnings projections. A few days later, Hanning obtains additional data that causes him to revise the projections downward. Right before public distribution of this report, Hanning learns that Jannsen has substituted the earlier, more favorable earnings projections into the report without Hanning's knowledge. Hanning should *most* appropriately:
   A. consult with internal counsel and insist that this matter be reported to the regulators immediately.
   B. insist that either the report be corrected, or his name be removed from the report.
   C. permit publication of this report, but issue a follow-up report correcting the earnings projections.

5. Andrew Pollard, CFA, overhears two executives from a multinational oil company discussing an unexpectedly large earnings increase the company is preparing to announce the following morning. When Pollard gets home that evening, he places an order to buy shares in this oil company. Which of the following *best* describes this situation?
   A. Pollard violated the Standards by acting on material nonpublic information.
   B. There is no violation of CFA Institute Standards, since this was simply an overheard conversation.
   C. Pollard violated CFA Institute Standards by not contacting counsel for advice before placing the trade.

6. Jim Whitaker is a director of an investment banking firm that is issuing a secondary offering for a company. The issue is oversubscribed. According to the firm's written trade allocation procedures, an oversubscribed issue must be distributed on a prorated basis among all interested clients. One of these clients is Whitaker himself. This procedure for allocating an oversubscribed issue is:
   A. in violation of the Standards because most clients will be receiving fewer shares than requested.
   B. in violation of the Standards because Whitaker should not participate if the issue is oversubscribed.
   C. not in violation of the Standards because all clients are treated fairly.

7. Morton Crane, CFA, is a portfolio manager. Crane has just been informed by his compliance officer that a new law will require additional disclosures of personal client information to regulators for two of Crane's former clients and one of his current clients. Crane decides to comply with the new law and provide the required client information. Has Crane violated CFA Institute Standards of Professional Conduct?
   A. No.
   B. Yes, because he disclosed confidential information about a former client.
   C. Yes, because he disclosed confidential information about a current client.

8. Telling potential investors that a short-term U.S. Treasury fund contains "guaranteed" securities:
   A. does not violate any Standard.
   B. violates the Standards by misrepresenting the securities in the fund.
   C. violates the Standards by failing to consider the suitability of the fund for potential investors.

9. A member provides a client with an investment performance presentation that does not include detailed information, but reflects the member's reasonable efforts to present results that are fair, accurate, and complete. Has the member complied with the Standard related to performance presentation?
   A. Yes, the member has met the requirements of the Standard.
   B. No, because the performance presentation must comply with Global Investment Performance Standards.
   C. No, because "reasonable efforts" do not ensure that the presentation is fair, accurate, and complete.

10. Isaac Jones, CFA, is a portfolio manager for a major brokerage firm. Jones wishes to buy Maxima common stock for some of his client's accounts. Jones also wishes to purchase Maxima for his personal account. In accordance with CFA Institute Standards, Jones may purchase Maxima for his personal account:
    A. only after completing the transactions for his clients.
    B. along with the purchases for his clients, as long as this is disclosed in advance to his clients and employer.
    C. at any time, as long as the execution price is not more favorable than the execution price received by the clients.

11. To comply with Global Investment Performance Standards (GIPS), a firm is *least likely* required to:
    A. provide a composite list and composite descriptions to any prospective client that requests them.
    B. hire an independent third-party verifier to prepare a report verifying the firm's GIPS compliance.
    C. provide a compliant presentation to all prospective clients.

12. The GIPS requirements regarding performance presentation of real estate investments:
    A. apply to most real estate investments, regardless of the degree of leverage or the degree of management by the firm.
    B. may or may not apply, depending on the level of control the firm has over the management of the investment.
    C. apply when leverage is involved in the real estate investment, but only for those real estate investments managed primarily by the firm.

13. Ken Howell, CFA, plans to issue a buy recommendation for Glazer Oil, Inc. based on his analysis and forecasts. Howell suspects that the company will soon announce merger plans with a Japanese oil company. To investigate, Howell attempts to call three executives at Glazer. Different secretaries inform Howell that the executives are "attending a conference overseas" or "traveling in Japan." Howell is able to confirm that all three are in the same city in Japan where the potential merger partner is headquartered. Howell feels confident that the merger will go forward. According to CFA Institute Standards of Professional Conduct, Howell may issue a buy recommendation on the oil company:
    A. immediately.
    B. only after allowing the companies a reasonable period of time to disclose their merger plans.
    C. only after urging the companies' managements to publicly disclose their merger plans.

14. Jerry Johnson, CFA, has been asked to write a research report on Luke's Lockers, a leading shoe manufacturer. Johnson's wife owns 5,000 shares of Luke's stock. To comply with the Code and Standards, Johnson's *most* appropriate action is to:
A. take no action since he does not own the stock directly.
B. disclose this ownership of the stock in the research report.
C. have his wife liquidate her holdings of the stock before the research report is released.

15. For the past five years, Rafael Garcia has served as a portfolio manager for Peak Investments. Garcia accepts a position at a competing firm. Garcia is not subject to a non-compete agreement. After beginning his new job, Garcia discovers files on his home computer that contain information about Peak's clients. Garcia shares this information with his new employer with the hope of bringing some of these clients over to his new firm. Garcia has:
A. violated the Standards because he has misused information belonging to Peak Investments.
B. not violated any Standards because he is permitted to contact former clients after he begins the new position.
C. not violated any Standard because he is not subject to a non-compete agreement.

16. In its initial GIPS-compliant performance presentation, a firm must show GIPS-compliant performance history for a:
A. minimum of five years or since firm's inception, and the firm must add annual performance results each year going forward for a minimum of five additional years of performance history.
B. maximum of five years or since firm's inception, and the firm must add annual performance results each year going forward up to a maximum of ten years of performance history.
C. minimum of five years or since firm's inception, and the firm must add annual performance results each year going forward up to a minimum total of ten years of performance history.

17. Randy Green, CFA, is a principal in an investment advisory firm. His firm has been retained by Bob Harris to manage a retirement fund of which Harris is a director. Green writes Harris a letter that states he will personally oversee the account and will always act in Harris's best interest. If Green acts in accordance with this statement, he will:
A. not violate the Code and Standards.
B. violate the Standard concering priority of transactions.
C. violate the Standard concering loyalty, prudence, and care.

18. James Bush, CFA, is meeting with an investor, George Stephan, for the first time. During their first meeting, Bush, before making any inquiry regarding the client's circumstances, outlines several investment strategies and also describes a specific stock with what Bush believes offers a high potential for large gains, and recommends that Stephan include this stock in his portfolio. With regard to suitability, Bush's actions:
A. comply with the Standards.
B. violate the Standards because Bush must determine Stephan's risk tolerance, objectives and needs before making any investment recommendations.
C. violate the Standards because Bush must obtain information on which securities the client has invested in previously, in order to make appropriate investment recommendations.

Questions 19 through 32 relate to Quantitative Methods. (21 minutes)

19. A brokerage company surveys 1,200 people at random to determine a relationship between age and participation in the stock market:

	Stock Trades Last Year	
Age	No	Yes
Under 30	325	235
Over 30	550	90

Based on the data from the survey, the empirical probability that a randomly chosen investor under the age of 30 made no stock trades in the last year is *closest* to:
A. 27%.
B. 31%.
C. 58%.

20. Lee Phillips, CFA, estimates that Biolab Inc. should earn $2.00 per share in 20X1, with a standard deviation of $1.00. If Biolab's earnings outcomes are normally distributed, the probability that Biolab earns $3.00 or more in 20X1 is *closest* to:
A. 16%.
B. 32%.
C. 34%.

21. An analyst has calculated the arithmetic, harmonic, and geometric mean using the last 10 years of returns on a stock. Which of these means should the analyst *most* appropriately use to forecast next year's return on the stock?
A. Harmonic mean.
B. Geometric mean.
C. Arithmetic mean.

22. The histogram of returns data for the Accel Equity Fund has a long left tail and is more peaked than a normal distribution. Based on the histogram, the distribution of returns for Accel has:
A. positive skewness.
B. negative skewness.
C. negative excess kurtosis.

23. Lisa McGrow, CFA, and Nelson Modello, CFA, are discussing alternative interpretations of interest rates. McGrow states that the opportunity cost of holding cash rises when interest rates rise. Modello states that the discounted value of a set of future cash flows rises when interest rates fall. Determine whether these statements are correct.
A. Both of these statements are correct.
B. Neither of these statements is correct.
C. Only one of these statements is correct.

24. Which of the following assumptions is *least* consistent with technical analysis?
A. Interaction of supply and demand causes trends in stock prices.
B. Information flow causes the market to reach a new equilibrium quickly.
C. Supply and demand is governed by both rational and irrational factors.

25. Seven of the twelve money managers employed by Hibbert Asset Management are eligible for a bonus, but only four bonuses are available. The bonuses vary in amounts, so the order in which they are awarded is important. The number of ways that Hibbert can award the bonuses is:
A. 28.
B. 210.
C. 840.

26. Ann Karson is evaluating a new drug product of Lancer Pharmaceutical Company. To receive approval, the new drug must reduce symptoms in a larger percentage of patients, on average, than the current standard of treatment. The *most* appropriate hypothesis test is a:
A. test of the population mean for the new drug.
B. test of differences between means of the new drug and current treatment.
C. paired comparisons test between the new drug and the current treatment.

27. For a two-tailed test of hypotheses on mean stock returns, using a 5% level of significance:
A. the null hypothesis should be rejected if the critical value for the test statistic exceeds the calculated value of the test statistic.
B. the null hypothesis should not be rejected if the hypothesized mean stock return lies within the 95% confidence interval.
C. the power of the test is the probability that the null hypothesis will not be rejected when it is true.

28. Jack Gallant lends €10,000 to his business partner Alex Wood. In exchange, Wood gives Gallant shares of preferred stock in MM Inc. paying €500 per year in dividends, and he agrees to repay €6,000 to Gallant at the end of year 1. The appropriate discount rate on the MM preferred shares is 10%. Gallant sells the MM preferred stock at the end of year 1, after receiving the first dividend. Gallant's 1-year holding period return is *closest* to:
A. 5%.
B. 10%.
C. 15%.

29. According to Elliott wave theory, an impulse wave is composed of:
A. five waves.
B. three waves.
C. five waves in an uptrend and three waves in a downtrend.

30. Kapila Securities provides brokerage and research services to high net worth clients. Kapila's research teams rank securities from one to five, with one representing "strong sell" and five representing "strong buy." The measurement scale that Kapila employs for securities rating is a(n):
A. ratio scale.
B. ordinal scale.
C. nominal scale.

31. According to the Central Limit Theorem:
    A. the distribution of sample means will be approximately normally distributed only if the population is normally distributed and continuous.
    B. inferences about the population mean can be made from the sample mean, as long as the sample size is sufficiently large.
    C. the sample mean will have a standard deviation equal to the population standard deviation divided by the sample size.

32. One of the major limitations of Monte Carlo simulation is that it:
    A. cannot provide the insight that analytic methods can.
    B. does not lend itself to performing "what if" scenarios.
    C. requires that variables be modeled using the normal distribution.

Questions 33 through 44 relate to Economics. (18 minutes)

33. A business believes a price discrimination strategy will increase both its output and profits. For this to occur, the firm must have:
    A. customers who cannot resell the product and whose price elasticities of demand are in a limited range.
    B. distinct groups of customers with different price elasticities of demand who are able to resell the product.
    C. distinct groups of customers with different price elasticities of demand who cannot resell the product.

34. John Bobson, CFA, states: "By imposing a tariff on a good, a country can increase its own economic welfare and, when the tariff revenue is included in the calculation, increase global economic welfare as well." Bobson's statement is:
    A. incorrect.
    B. correct, if the country is a large importer of the good.
    C. correct, if the country is a large exporter of the good.

35. Functions of a central bank *most likely* include:
    A. collecting tax payments.
    B. balancing the national budget.
    C. controlling money supply growth.

36. An increase in oil prices reduces short-run aggregate supply. Real GDP decreases and the price level increases. The central bank responds by increasing the money supply to increase aggregate demand and restore full employment. Further increases in oil prices require repeated action by the central bank. This is an example of:
    A. an inflationary gap.
    B. cost-push inflation.
    C. demand-pull inflation

37. Assume a cartel is organized among the producers of a commodity and begins practicing collusion. The *most likely* effects on price and output are that:
A. both will increase.
B. price will increase and output will decrease.
C. price will decrease and output will increase.

38. Long-run aggregate supply is *most likely* to increase as a result of a(n):
A. increase in expected inflation.
B. decrease in the real wage rate.
C. increase in aggregate hours worked.

39. The velocity of transactions in an economy has been increasing rapidly for the past seven years. Over the same time period, the economy has experienced minimal growth in real output. According to the equation of exchange, inflation over the last seven years has:
A. increased more than the growth in the money supply.
B. been minimal, consistent with the slow growth in real output.
C. increased at a rate similar to the growth rate in the money supply.

40. Average total costs for Dunhill Corporation's turbine plant are minimized when production is 100,000 units per year. Justin Collins states that (1) average variable cost is minimized at this same level of production, and that (2) profit is maximized at this level of production. Are Collins' statements accurate?
A. Both statements are accurate.
B. Neither statement is accurate.
C. Only one of the statements is accurate.

41. The market supply function for a good is $Q_S = -120 + 5P$ and the market demand function for the good is $Q_D = 440 - 9P$. If the price of the good is 45, competitive forces will:
A. increase the price and increase the quantity supplied.
B. increase the price and decrease the quantity demanded.
C. decrease the price and increase the quantity demanded.

42. When arbitrage trading is able to take place, the difference between the spot and forward exchange rates for a pair of currencies is *most likely* to reflect the difference between the two countries' domestic:
A. growth rates.
B. interest rates.
C. inflation rates.

43. Which of the following arguments about the efficiency of monopolistic competition in allocating resources is *most* accurate?
    A. Since economic profits in the long run are positive for firms in monopolistic competition, there are efficiency losses.
    B. Product differentiation under monopolistic competition offers benefits that tend to offset inefficiency from the reduction in output compared to perfect competition.
    C. Advertising expenditures under monopolistic competition represent a deadweight loss to society.

44. A firm faces a downward sloping demand curve, $Q_D = 500 - 20P$. The marginal revenue if the price were decreased from \$18.00 to \$17.95 is *closest* to:
    A. \$11.
    B. \$13.
    C. \$15.

Questions 45 through 68 relate to Financial Reporting and Analysis. (36 minutes)

45. Rossdale, Inc., buys a small manufacturing plant with an estimated useful life of 12 years. The building includes two built-in machines that are expected to be replaced after four years and six years. Under International Financial Reporting Standards, Rossdale:
    A. must have a single depreciation schedule for the plant.
    B. may have separate depreciation schedules for the machines and the building.
    C. must have separate depreciation schedules for the machines and the building.

46. A firm's balance sheet is *most likely* to reflect the value of a firm's:
    A. brand names.
    B. operating leases.
    C. investments in derivatives.

47. A company understates year-end depreciation. As compared to the properly stated year-end results, what effect will this understatement have on the company's asset turnover ratio?
    A. No impact.
    B. Decrease.
    C. Increase.

48. A manufacturing company reports research costs and a loss on the sale of a business segment on its income statement. Which of these items should be included in operating expenses?
    A. Neither of these items.
    B. Only one of these items.
    C. Both of these items.

49. Thunderbird Company reported net income of $500 million and the company had 100 million common shares outstanding. In addition, Thunderbird had 5 million shares of convertible preferred and 10 million outstanding warrants during the year. Each preferred share pays a dividend of $4 per share and is convertible into three common shares. Each warrant is convertible into one common share at $25 per share. The company's stock traded at an average $50 per share. Thunderbird's diluted earnings per share for the year is *closest* to:
    A. $4.00 per share.
    B. $4.20 per share.
    C. $4.80 per share.

50. An analyst would *most likely* suspect that the quality of a company's earnings is deteriorating if the company:
    A. has a cash flow earnings index greater than one.
    B. increases the estimated useful lives and salvage values of several physical assets.
    C. classifies the lease of a machine the company will employ for 50% of its estimated useful life as an operating lease.

51. Under U.S. GAAP, how is goodwill related to an acquisition measured and shown on the acquirer's financial statements following the acquisition?
    A. Measured at excess of purchase cost over the fair value of the assets at acquisition date and recorded as an intangible asset.
    B. Measured at present value of future estimated excess cash flows from the acquisition and recorded as an intangible asset.
    C. Not recorded as an asset, but the present value of future estimated excess cash flows is disclosed in the financial statement notes.

52. A company's investments in marketable securities include actively traded equity securities, long-term bonds available for sale, and long-term bonds held to maturity.

	Stock Held for Trading	*Bonds Available for Sale*	*Bonds Held to Maturity*
Change in market value	$200,000 increase	$100,000 decrease	No change
Dividend and interest income	$30,000	$50,000	$10,000

Taken together, these investments increase the company's pretax income by:
A. $90,000.
B. $190,000.
C. $290,000.

53. The role of financial statement analysis is *best* described as:
A. a common requirement for companies that are listed on public exchanges.
B. the reports and presentations a company uses to show its financial performance to investors, creditors, and other interested parties.
C. the use of information from a company's financial statements along with other information to make economic decisions regarding that company.

54. During 20X1, Tusa Company sold machinery with an original cost of \$100,000, and recognized a \$15,000 gain from the sale. At the time of the sale, the accumulated depreciation of the machinery was \$80,000. Ignoring taxes, the machinery sale will produce a:
A. \$15,000 inflow from investing activities.
B. \$20,000 inflow from operating activities.
C. \$35,000 inflow from investing activities.

55. David Chance, CFA, is analyzing Grow Corporation. Chance gathers the following information:

Net cash provided by operating activities	\$3,500
Net cash used for fixed capital investments	\$727
Cash paid for interest	\$195
Income before tax	\$4,400
Income tax expense	\$1,540
Net income	\$2,860

Grow's free cash flow to the firm (FCFF) is *closest* to:
A. \$2,260.
B. \$2,640.
C. \$2,900.

56. For the last few years, firms in an expanding industry have found it more difficult to keep up with consumer demand despite steadily increasing inventory levels. The Consumer Price Index (CPI) has been at a level of 1050, 1060, and 1087 in the last three years. Given this situation, a firm in this industry that seeks to report higher net income would *most likely* prefer which inventory accounting method?
A. LIFO.
B. FIFO.
C. Average cost.

57. Cheryl Flynn, CFA, is preparing her recommendation for the stock of Garrett Company. Flynn believes Garrett's reported sales are of poor quality because its managers recognize revenue too aggressively. To show that her opinion has a reasonable basis, Flynn is *least likely* to:
A. compare relevant financial statement data and ratios for Garrett to those of other firms in its industry.
B. examine the disclosures of significant accounting policies that are included with Garrett's financial statements.
C. contrast the billings and collections on Garrett's general ledger with the amounts reported on its financial statements.

58. A lessee has an incentive to report a lease as an operating lease rather than a finance lease because in the initial period, reporting a lease as an operating lease, rather than as a finance lease, will result in:
A. greater total cash flow.
B. higher operating income.
C. a lower debt-to-equity ratio.

59. Mustang Corporation acquired Cobra Company five years ago. As a part of the acquisition, Mustang reported goodwill of $750,000. For the year just ended, Mustang gathered the following data:

• Fair value of Cobra	$5,000,000
• Carrying value of Cobra (including goodwill)	$5,200,000
• Identifiable net assets of Cobra at fair value	$4,500,000

Using U.S. GAAP, the goodwill is:
A. impaired and a loss of $200,000 is recognized.
B. impaired and a loss of $250,000 is recognized.
C. not impaired and no loss is recognized.

60. POI Corp. has an effective tax rate of 29.6% and a statutory tax rate of 35%. The cause of this difference is *most likely*:
A. warranty expense.
B. accelerated depreciation.
C. permanently reinvested earnings of a foreign subsidiary.

61. Use of the indirect method of presenting cash flows from operating activities:
A. is encouraged by both the IASB and FASB.
B. illustrates the reasons for the difference between net income and operating cash flow.
C. requires disclosure of the cash flows that would be presented using the direct method.

62. Hazel Edwards, CFA, is analyzing Collins Footwear, Inc. and obtains the following data for the company's major geographic segments:

	Asia	*Europe*	*North America*
Sales (U.S. dollars)	$200 million	$300 million	$500 million
Net profit margin	4.5%	3.0%	1.5%
Asset turnover	1.5×	2.5×	4.0×

Based on these data, Edwards should conclude that Collins's:
A. smallest segment by assets is Asia.
B. most profitable segment by return on assets is Europe.
C. most profitable segment by net income is North America.

63. Shelby Enterprises recently entered into a new $500 million revolving credit facility. The provisions of the facility require Shelby to repay the loan before any other debt can be retired. In addition, if the company's debt-to-capital ratio is higher than 1.0 or their equity falls below $2 billion, Shelby will be prohibited from paying any dividends. Shelby would *most likely* agree to these covenants because they reduce:
A. risk to bondholders.
B. the company's interest cost.
C. risk to shareholders.

64. Selected information on Reckner Company's income taxes appears in the following table:

	20X1	*20X2*	*20X3*
Taxes payable	250	500	500
Deferred tax assets	200	300	200
Deferred tax liabilities	200	300	400

Compared to 20X2, Reckner's 20X3 income tax expense:
A. increased.
B. decreased.
C. remained the same.

65. On December 31, Pinto Company redeems its $1,000,000, 8% bonds at 101% of par and reports an extraordinary loss of $12,000. Assuming Pinto's tax rate is 40%, what is the carrying value of the bonds on the call date?
A. $990,000.
B. $998,000.
C. $1,030,000.

66. Under which accounting standards *must* a company recognize construction interest as an expense?
A. IFRS, but not U.S. GAAP.
B. U.S. GAAP, but not IFRS.
C. Neither IFRS nor U.S. GAAP.

67. At the end of last year, Manhattan Corporation had a quick ratio of 1.2. If Manhattan reduces its accounts payable with a cash payment of $2 million, its quick ratio will:
A. be unchanged.
B. increase.
C. decrease.

68. An analyst gathers the following selected financial information on Quip Corp.

Partial financials for 20X8	*Quip Corp*
Sales	$350,000
Cost of goods sold	270,000
Net income	35,000
Current assets	165,000
Current liabilities	130,000
20X8 LIFO reserve	30,000
20X7 LIFO reserve	20,000

To compare Quip and its competitors, an analyst makes the necessary adjustments to restate Quip's financial statements to reflect the FIFO inventory accounting method. Quip's adjusted gross profit margin is *closest* to:
A. 20%.
B. 23%.
C. 26%.

Questions 69 through 78 relate to Corporate Finance. (15 minutes)

69. A company's excess cash balances can *most* appropriately be invested in:
A. common stock.
B. corporate bonds.
C. commercial paper.

70. Paola Antolini, CFA, has been nominated to serve on the board of directors of CoMedia, an entertainment conglomerate. Antolini's experience *most likely* qualifies her to serve the best interests of CoMedia's shareowners if she:
A. served on the board of a pharmaceutical company for the past eight years.
B. has a longstanding professional relationship with several CoMedia executives.
C. adheres to a policy of not owning shares of companies for which she serves as a director.

71. A guarantee stating that a payment will be made upon receipt of goods or services is *best* known as:
A. commercial paper.
B. a banker's acceptance.
C. a revolving line of credit.

72. Inverness Corporation is considering investing in one of two mutually exclusive capital projects. The firm's cost of capital is 15%. Project A's NPV profile crosses the Y-axis at $1.8 million and crosses the X-axis at 25%. Project B's NPV profile crosses the Y-axis at $1.2 million and crosses the X-axis at 33%. For the two projects the crossover rate is 18%. Which of the following is *most likely* correct?
A. Project A and Project B have equal NPVs at a discount rate of 15%.
B. Inverness should choose Project B since it has a higher IRR.
C. Inverness should choose Project A since it has a higher NPV.

73. Benson Inc. has a number of company policies that affect shareholder rights. Which of Benson's policies is *most likely* to be considered as not in the shareholders' best interests?
A. Benson requires two-thirds majority shareholder approval for any takeover defense proposed by the firm's managers.
B. Benson's board of directors tabulates the results of all proxy votes, which are recorded and maintained by an independent third party.
C. Benson has two classes of common shares. Each Class 2 share has one-tenth the ownership interest and one-tenth the voting power of a Class 1 share.

74. The effects that the acceptance of a project may have on other firm cash flows are *best* described as:
A. pure plays.
B. externalities.
C. opportunity costs.

75. Compared to retaining 100% of net income, paying a cash dividend results in:
    A. higher financial leverage ratios and lower liquidity ratios.
    B. lower liquidity ratios and no effect on financial leverage ratios.
    C. lower financial leverage ratios and no effect on liquidity ratios.

76. While analyzing HMS Inc., Fred Browne notes that the company's liquidity as measured by its quick ratio has decreased over time while its current liabilities have remained constant. This could be explained by a(n):
    A. decrease in inventory.
    B. increase in marketable securities.
    C. decrease in accounts receivable.

77. With regard to the internal rate of return (IRR), which of the following statements is *most* accurate?
    A. The IRR is the discount rate that maximizes a project's net present value.
    B. A proper decision rule is to accept the project if IRR is less than the required rate of return.
    C. IRR is the discount rate at which the present value of expected future after-tax cash flows is equal to the investment outlay.

78. Walker Company plans to borrow $25 million to repurchase 5% of its 10 million outstanding shares at the market price of $50. Walker's earnings per share before the repurchase are $2.00. If walker's after-tax cost of debt is 4%, what effect will the share repurchase have on its earnings per share? The share repurchase will:
    A. increase earnings per share.
    B. decrease earnings per share.
    C. have no effect on earnings per share.

Questions 79 through 84 relate to Portfolio Management. (9 minutes)

79. A risk-averse investor prefers the lowest-risk investment:
    A. for any given level of expected return.
    B. when presented with three investment alternatives.
    C. with an expected return at least equal to her threshold rate of return.

80. The execution step in the portfolio management process is *most likely* to include:
    A. asset allocation and security analysis.
    B. preparation of an investment policy statement.
    C. performance measurement and portfolio rebalancing.

81. Which of the following portfolio constraints in the Investment Policy Statement of a local college's endowment *most likely* belongs in the "unique needs and preferences" category? The endowment is:
A. exempt from taxes.
B. subject to oversight by a regulatory authority.
C. unwilling to invest in companies that sell weapons.

82. Adding the risk-free asset to a portfolio of risky assets will:
A. decrease portfolio standard deviation because it is uncorrelated with risky assets.
B. not affect portfolio standard deviation because it is uncorrelated with risky assets.
C. decrease portfolio standard deviation due to its negative correlation with risky assets.

83. An investor buys a non-dividend paying stock for $100 at the beginning of the year with 50% initial margin. At the end of the year, the stock price is $95. Deflation of 2% occurred during the year. Which of the following return measures for this investment will be greatest?
A. Real return.
B. Nominal return.
C. Leveraged return.

84. Penny Linn, CFA, predicts that both Stock X and Y will return 20% next year. The Treasury bill rate is 5% and the market risk premium is 8%. The beta for Stock X is 1.5 and for Stock Y is 2. The standard deviation for Stock X is 20% and for Stock Y is 30%. Linn believes that:
A. Stock X is overvalued and Stock Y is undervalued.
B. Stock X is undervalued and Stock Y is overvalued.
C. Both Stock X and Stock Y are overvalued.

Questions 85 through 96 relate to Equity Investments. (18 minutes)

85. Jacques Fontenot wants to place an order to purchase 10,000 shares of BQ Inc. at a price of €75.00 or below. The shares are currently trading for €82.10 bid and €82.20 ask. What type of order should Fontenot place?
A. Market order.
B. Stop loss order.
C. Limit order.

86. With respect to a well-functioning securities market, a market that exhibits operational efficiency will have:
A. price continuity.
B. low transaction costs.
C. rapid price reactions to new information.

87. An investor owns preference shares which stipulate that any dividend for the current period, as well as all past dividends, must be fully paid before a common stock dividend may be paid. This security is *best* described as:
A. full-pay preferred.
B. restricted preferred.
C. cumulative preferred.

88. For the year 20X5, Felden Company's book value of equity increased by 4% while its market value of equity decreased by 2%. Based only on this information, it is *most likely* that:
A. Felden carried out a 1-for-2 reverse stock split.
B. investors reduced their expectations about Felden's future cash flows.
C. Felden repurchased a portion of its common stock for cash at the market price.

89. Larry Rile is evaluating the investment merits of Bing Corp., a successful motorcycle manufacturer. Rile is forecasting a dividend in year 1 of $1.50 per share, a dividend in year 2 of $3.00 per share, and a dividend in year 3 of $4.50 per share. After year 3, Rile expects dividends to grow at the rate of 6% per year. Rile calculates a beta of 1.3 for Bing. Rile expects the S&P 500 index to return 8%. The U.S. Treasury bill is yielding 2%. Using the multistage dividend discount model, Bing's intrinsic value is *closest* to:
A. $92 per share.
B. $102 per share.
C. $112 per share.

90. Ian Lance, CFA, is discussing short selling with a client and states, "The short seller must pay any dividend to the lender of the stock. In addition, the short seller must provide collateral to the brokerage house." Has Lance stated the short seller's obligations accurately?
A. Both of these statements are accurate.
B. Neither of these statements is accurate.
C. Only one of these statements is accurate.

91. Enterprise value is *most accurately* interpreted as the:
A. cost to take over a firm.
B. fair market value of a firm's equity.
C. market value of a firm's equity plus the market value of its debt.

92. Given the academic research supporting the efficiency of the stock market, which of the following is the *least accurate* description of a portfolio manager's role in an efficient market?
A. Identifying and specifying a client's objectives and constraints.
B. Specifying an explicit investment strategy to meet the client's needs.
C. Diversifying the client's portfolio across all asset classes to eliminate systematic risk.

93. Compared with publicly traded firms, private equity firms *most likely* tend to:
A. focus more on long-term performance.
B. adopt stronger corporate governance policies.
C. be more closely regulated and have higher compliance costs.

94. A firm attempts to gain market share from its competitors by improving its manufacturing efficiency so that it can increase output and reduce the price of its product. This firm's competitive strategy is *most accurately* described as a(n):
A. offensive differentiation strategy.
B. offensive cost leadership strategy.
C. defensive cost leadership strategy.

95. A multi-market index is *most likely* to overweight countries that have recently experienced high equity market returns if it weights the securities in each country index by:
A. dividend yield, and weights the country index returns by market capitalization.
B. dividend yield, and weights the country index returns by gross domestic product.
C. market capitalization, and weights the country index returns by gross domestic product.

96. In valuing the stock of Evergreen Enterprises, an analyst compiles the following information about the firm:

Expected constant growth rate of dividends	6%
Next year's expected earnings per share	$4.24
Expected retention ratio	62.5%
Required rate of return	11%

The value of the firm's stock today is *closest* to:
A. $31.80.
B. $38.55.
C. $53.00.

Questions 97 through 110 relate to Fixed Income. (21 minutes)

97. An analyst is evaluating an annual-pay bond with a yield to maturity of 7.0%. The bond-equivalent yield of this bond is:
    A. equal to 7.0%.
    B. less than 7.0%.
    C. greater than 7.0%.

98. An economist has forecast that the term structure of interest rates will remain flat. According to the liquidity preference theory, the economist's forecast implies that future short-term interest rates will:
    A. decrease over time.
    B. increase over time.
    C. equal current short-term interest rates.

99. For institutional investors financing bond purchases:
    A. repurchase agreements usually offer lower interest costs than margin buying.
    B. margin buying usually allows for borrowing a higher percentage of the collateral value than a repurchase agreement.
    C. margin buying is usually the preferred transaction structure.

100. Eric Webb, an individual investor in a high tax bracket, would like to purchase a 5-year zero-coupon security with no credit risk. His investment adviser has recommended U.S. Treasury STRIP securities, and has told Webb that either coupon STRIPs or principal STRIPs would meet his needs. The adviser should also inform Webb that:
    A. while principal STRIPs have no credit risk, there is credit risk in coupon STRIPs.
    B. principal STRIPs have higher reinvestment risk than the coupon STRIPs.
    C. investing in STRIP securities may have adverse tax consequences.

101. Tunopani is an emerging market nation that issues sovereign debt denominated in its local currency and sovereign debt denominated in a developed market currency. If Tunopani's local currency debt rating is A2/A, its foreign currency debt rating is *most likely* to be:
    A. lower.
    B. higher.
    C. the same.

102. An analyst states that the purpose of a collateralized mortgage obligation is to redistribute prepayment risk among investors with different risk tolerances while reducing total prepayment risk for all tranches in the structure. The analyst's statement is correct:
A. only with respect to redistribution of risk.
B. only with respect to reducing total prepayment risk.
C. with respect to both redistribution of risk and reducing total prepayment risk.

103. Jorge Fullen is evaluating a 7%, 10-year bond that is callable at par in 5 years. Coupon payments can be reinvested at an annual rate of 7%, and the current price of the bond is $106.50. The bond pays interest semiannually. Should Fullen consider the yield to first call (YTC) or the yield to maturity (YTM) in making his purchase decision?
A. YTM, since YTM is greater than YTC.
B. YTC, since YTC is less than YTM.
C. YTC, since YTC is greater than YTM.

104. PRC International just completed a $234 million floating rate convertible bond offering. As stated in the indenture, the interest rate on the bond is the lesser of 90-day LIBOR or 10%. The indenture also requires PRC to retire $5.6 million per year with the option to retire as much as $10 million. Which of the following embedded options is *most likely* to benefit the investor? The:
A. 10% cap on the floating interest rate.
B. accelerated sinking fund provision for principal repayment.
C. conversion option on the convertible bonds.

105. An advantage of the duration/convexity approach over the full valuation approach is:
A. its superior accuracy for nonparallel shifts in the yield curve.
B. it is not based on yield to maturity, which is a summary measure.
C. it saves considerable time when working with portfolios of bonds.

106. Siegel, Inc. has issued bonds maturing in 15 years but callable at any time after the first 8 years. The bonds have a coupon rate of 6%, and are currently trading at $992 per $1,000 par value. If interest rates decline over the next few years:
A. the call option embedded in the bonds will increase in value, but the price of the bond will decrease.
B. the price of the bond will increase, but probably by less than a comparable bond with no embedded option.
C. the price of the bond will increase, primarily as a result of the increasing value of the call option.

107. Bond X carries a rating of BBB-/Baa3. Bond Y has a rating of B/B2. Both bonds mature in ten years. Which bond's value would be *most* affected by a ratings downgrade, and which bond has the higher default risk?
   A. Bond X would be more affected by a ratings downgrade, but Bond Y has higher default risk.
   B. Bond Y would be more affected by a ratings downgrade, but Bond X has higher default risk.
   C. Bond X has higher default risk, but both bonds would experience similar effects of a ratings downgrade.

108. Karen Callaway is an investor in the 35% tax bracket. She is evaluating a tax-exempt municipal security with a tax-exempt yield of 4.5%. What is the taxable equivalent yield of the municipal security?
   A. 2.9%.
   B. 6.9%.
   C. 12.9%.

109. Ron Logan, CFA, is a bond manager. He purchased $50 million in 6.0% coupon Southwest Manufacturing bonds at par three years ago. Today, the bonds are priced to yield 6.85%. The bonds mature in nine years. The Southwest bonds are trading at a:
   A. discount, and the yield to maturity has increased since purchase.
   B. premium, and the yield to maturity has decreased since purchase.
   C. discount and the yield to maturity has decreased since purchase.

110. Six-month LIBOR is an interest rate which:
   A. represents the interest rate paid on a CD that matures in 6 months.
   B. is the return available on the shortest term euro-denominated securities.
   C. is determined by adding a small spread to the yield available on a UK government bond maturing in 6 months.

Questions 111 through 116 relate to Derivatives. (9 minutes)

111. Two portfolio managers are discussing option strategies. Connie Solis, CFA, states that a covered call strategy preserves the upside potential from appreciation in the underlying stock, while reducing the downside risk. Lou Millwood, CFA, states that a protective put strategy has unlimited upside potential, with potential losses limited to an amount equal to the stock price minus the put premium. Are these statements accurate?
   A. Both of these statements are accurate.
   B. Neither of these statements is accurate.
   C. Only one of these statements is accurate.

112. Sally Ferguson, CFA, is a hedge fund manager. Ferguson utilizes both futures and forward contracts in the fund she manages. Ferguson makes the following statements about futures and forward contracts:

Statement 1: A futures contract is an exchange traded instrument with standardized features.

Statement 2: Forward contracts are marked to market on a daily basis to reduce credit risk to both counterparties.

Are Ferguson's statements accurate?
A. Both of these statements are accurate.
B. Neither of these statements is accurate.
C. Only one of these statements is accurate.

113. Anne Quincy took the short side of a forward contract on the S&P 500 Index three months ago in an attempt to hedge short-term changes in her index portfolio. The contract had a term of six months at the purchase date, a contract price of $1,221 and Mason Inc. as the counterparty. Quincy is now considering unwinding her short position using either a three-month Mason Inc. contract with a price of $1,220, a three-month JonesCo contract with a price of $1,219, or a three-month Redding Company contract with a price of $1,218. If Quincy wants to minimize credit risk, she should take the long position in the contract with:
A. JonesCo.
B. Mason Inc.
C. Redding Company.

114. An analyst is evaluating a European call option with a strike price of 25 and 219 days to expiration. The underlying stock is currently trading for $29. If the risk-free rate is 4.0%, what is the lower bound on the value of this option?
A. $0.
B. $4.00.
C. $4.58.

115. Chris Kramer holds three options that expire on the same day. Option 1 is a call option on the stock of Blintz Company with a strike price of $58. Option 2 is an interest rate put option on 90-day LIBOR with a strike price of 5.4% and notional principal of $1,000. Option 3 is a put option on InstaCare stock with a strike price of $23. On the expiration date of the options, if the price of Blintz stock is $64, 90-day LIBOR is 3.0%, and the price of InstaCare stock is $29, Kramer will receive the largest cash flow from:
A. Option 1.
B. Option 2.
C. Option 3.

116. Phil Anderson, CFA, enters into a plain vanilla 1-year interest rate swap agreement with Baker Bank in which he will make fixed-rate payments in exchange for receiving floating-rate payments based on LIBOR plus 100 basis points. Assume that payments are made quarterly in arrears based on a 360-day year. The fixed rate on the swap is 6.5%. The current interest rates on 90, 180, and 360-day LIBOR are 5.2%, 5.5%, and 6.0%, respectively. If the notional principal is $100 million, Anderson's net cash flow at the end of the first quarter will equal:
A. –$675,000.
B. –$75,000.
C. +$75,000.

Questions 117 through 120 relate to Alternative Investments. (6 minutes)

117. A hedge fund that engages primarily in distressed debt investing and merger arbitrage is *best* described as using a(n):
A. macro strategy.
B. event-driven strategy.
C. relative value strategy.

118. The period of time during which a private equity fund will select investments and direct committed capital to them is *best* described as a:
A. notice period.
B. lockup period.
C. drawdown period.

119. A long-only commodity index investment is *most likely*:
A. to perform poorly in inflationary periods.
B. considered a passive investment strategy.
C. to be implemented by using derivatives.

120. Assume most hedge funds have a 2-and-20 fee structure and most funds of funds have a 1-and-10 fee structure. Over a long investment horizon, compared to net returns from investing directly in hedge funds, net returns from investing in funds of funds are *most likely* to be:
A. lower.
B. higher.
C. the same.

End of Morning Session

Exam 3
Afternoon Session

Topic	Questions	Points
Ethical and Professional Standards	1–18	27
Quantitative Methods	19–32	21
Economics	33–44	18
Financial Reporting and Analysis	45–68	36
Corporate Finance	69–78	15
Portfolio Management	79–84	9
Equity Investments	85–96	18
Fixed Income	97–110	21
Derivatives	111–116	9
Alternative Investments	117–120	6
Total		**180**

Test Answers

1.	A	B	C	41.	A	B	C	81.	A	B	C
2.	A	B	C	42.	A	B	C	82.	A	B	C
3.	A	B	C	43.	A	B	C	83.	A	B	C
4.	A	B	C	44.	A	B	C	84.	A	B	C
5.	A	B	C	45.	A	B	C	85.	A	B	C
6.	A	B	C	46.	A	B	C	86.	A	B	C
7.	A	B	C	47.	A	B	C	87.	A	B	C
8.	A	B	C	48.	A	B	C	88.	A	B	C
9.	A	B	C	49.	A	B	C	89.	A	B	C
10.	A	B	C	50.	A	B	C	90.	A	B	C
11.	A	B	C	51.	A	B	C	91.	A	B	C
12.	A	B	C	52.	A	B	C	92.	A	B	C
13.	A	B	C	53.	A	B	C	93.	A	B	C
14.	A	B	C	54.	A	B	C	94.	A	B	C
15.	A	B	C	55.	A	B	C	95.	A	B	C
16.	A	B	C	56.	A	B	C	96.	A	B	C
17.	A	B	C	57.	A	B	C	97.	A	B	C
18.	A	B	C	58.	A	B	C	98.	A	B	C
19.	A	B	C	59.	A	B	C	99.	A	B	C
20.	A	B	C	60.	A	B	C	100.	A	B	C
21.	A	B	C	61.	A	B	C	101.	A	B	C
22.	A	B	C	62.	A	B	C	102.	A	B	C
23.	A	B	C	63.	A	B	C	103.	A	B	C
24.	A	B	C	64.	A	B	C	104.	A	B	C
25.	A	B	C	65.	A	B	C	105.	A	B	C
26.	A	B	C	66.	A	B	C	106.	A	B	C
27.	A	B	C	67.	A	B	C	107.	A	B	C
28.	A	B	C	68.	A	B	C	108.	A	B	C
29.	A	B	C	69.	A	B	C	109.	A	B	C
30.	A	B	C	70.	A	B	C	110.	A	B	C
31.	A	B	C	71.	A	B	C	111.	A	B	C
32.	A	B	C	72.	A	B	C	112.	A	B	C
33.	A	B	C	73.	A	B	C	113.	A	B	C
34.	A	B	C	74.	A	B	C	114.	A	B	C
35.	A	B	C	75.	A	B	C	115.	A	B	C
36.	A	B	C	76.	A	B	C	116.	A	B	C
37.	A	B	C	77.	A	B	C	117.	A	B	C
38.	A	B	C	78.	A	B	C	118.	A	B	C
39.	A	B	C	79.	A	B	C	119.	A	B	C
40.	A	B	C	80.	A	B	C	120.	A	B	C

Exam 3
Afternoon Session

Questions 1 through 18 relate to Ethical and Professional Standards. (27 minutes)

1. Ray Brown, CFA, gives prospects his firm's marketing materials, not prepared by him, that indicate he has a graduate degree from State University, when in fact he did graduate work there but did not receive a degree. Brown informed the marketing department of this error when he first saw it. Brown has:
   A. violated the Standards by misrepresenting his qualifications.
   B. not violated the Standards because he has informed his firm of the mistake.
   C. not violated the Standards because he did not prepare the marketing materials or misrepresent his credentials to his firm.

2. John Larsen, CFA, is creating his investment firm's initial GIPS-compliant performance results. He would like to supplement the historical performance numbers with older, non-GIPS-compliant data. According to GIPS, is this allowed?
   A. GIPS results cannot include presentation of any noncompliant performance data.
   B. After the initial, GIPS-compliant performance results are presented, a firm may go back further and present non-compliant performance data, but no non-compliant results can be included for time periods after January 1, 2000.
   C. As long as five years of GIPS-compliant performance results are presented, the firm can go back further and present non-compliant performance data.

3. A member or candidate who changes his recommendation on a stock can comply with the Standards by communicating this change to clients according to:
   A. size of the client.
   B. known interest of the client in the stock.
   C. number of shares of the stock owned by the client.

4. Lyndon Westerburg, CFA, manages individual accounts. One of his clients offers Westerburg use of his yacht for a week if the client's portfolio exceeds specified benchmarks. Westerburg discloses this to his employer and obtains permission to accept the arrangement. Is Westerburg in compliance with CFA Institute Standards of Professional Conduct?
   A. This is a violation of CFA Institute Standards because Westerburg did not disclose the additional compensation to the other clients.
   B. Westerburg has violated the independence and objectivity Standard by accepting a substantial gift which could compromise his independence and objectivity.
   C. No violation of the Standards has occurred.

5. Rob Carter, CFA, is preparing a research report on Clean Bright, a company that manufactures cleaning products. After reviewing industry statistics and consulting with several suppliers of Clean Bright, Carter discovers that Clean Bright has become alarmingly slow in meeting its accounts payable. Carter believes that the company may soon face bankruptcy. Before Carter can issue a sell recommendation in his research report, Carter is required to:
   A. take no additional action, and can freely issue the report.
   B. wait until suppliers contact other analysts about Clean Bright.
   C. make full disclosure of the conversations with the suppliers to a compliance officer at his firm.

6. To comply with GIPS, private equity investments must be valued according to specific guidelines contained in Appendix D, the "GIPS Private Equity Valuation Principles." Exceptions, in which private equity investments can be valued according to the main body of GIPS, include:
   A. evergreen funds and open-end funds.
   B. closed-end funds and venture capital investments.
   C. venture capital investments and mezzanine financing.

7. Harriet Kedzie, CFA, manages a portfolio for a foundation. In a recent report to the foundation's directors, Kedzie explained her rationale for investing in ZYX stock as follows: "ZYX was chosen since it further diversifies the Foundation's holdings without sacrificing expected returns. In fact, ZYX's low standard deviation and high expected return ensure that the foundation will benefit from positive returns on this investment." Kedzie has *most likely*:
   A. not violated any Standards.
   B. violated the Standard concerning suitability.
   C. violated the Standard concerning misrepresentation.

8. Ken Koski, CFA, issues a press release that includes the following statement:

> "We are proud to announce that two of our managers have earned the right to use the CFA designation. In addition, four of our junior analysts have become Level III CFA candidates. These individuals have proven their dedication to the investment community and shown commitment to the highest ethical standards."

With regard to the statements in the press release:
A. all these statements are in compliance with CFA Institute Standards.
B. Koski has violated the Code and Standards by improperly referencing the managers' right to use the CFA designation.
C. Koski has violated the Code and Standards by implying superior performance results.

9. Which of the following statements *best* describes how GIPS requires portfolios to be grouped into composites?
A. Composites can include model results, if this is clearly specified.
B. All discretionary portfolios must be included in at least one composite if they are still managed by the firm.
C. Each composite must include all discretionary portfolios that the firm has managed according to that particular composite strategy or style, including closed accounts.

10. With regard to independent practice by Members and Candidates who are employed, the Code and Standards specify that:
A. undertaking independent practice includes preparations to begin such practice.
B. written consent must be obtained from both the employer and clients who may be affected.
C. members and candidates contemplating independent competitive business must notify their current employer of the types of services to be rendered, duration, and compensation.

11. Doug Watson is a senior portfolio manager for Pinnacle Capital. Pinnacle currently holds a substantial position in ATI Corporation, a large oil and gas exploration company. ATI's managers visit Pinnacle's offices to give their financial presentation. After the presentation, ATI's president mentions to Watson that he believes ATI is on the verge of a major natural gas discovery in Texas. News of this potential financial windfall had not been mentioned during the presentation. To comply with CFA Institute Standards of Professional Conduct, Watson should:
A. encourage the president of ATI to make the information public.
B. communicate the information to Pinnacle's designated compliance officer before trading or causing others to trade on it.
C. prohibit all trading of ATI by Pinnacle until the information is publicly disseminated.

12. Wally Manaugh, CFA, rates BriteCo as a "hold." He meets with other analysts in a social context and overhears a group talking favorably about BriteCo. He believes one of the group members is a former employee of BriteCo. Upon returning to his office, he second-guesses his initial analysis and tilts his report to be a bit more favorable, although he retains the "hold" recommendation. Manaugh has *most likely* violated the Standards because he:
    A. cannot trade or cause others to trade on this information.
    B. does not have a reasonable and adequate basis to change his report.
    C. failed to distinguish fact from opinion.

13. Martin Remy, CFA, has a client who says she expects a large inheritance soon that she will need to invest. Remy contacts Johan Walker, who handles the fixed-income portion of the client's portfolio, and informs him about the inheritance. Walker tells Remy that based on suspicious activity in the client's account, he suspects the inheritance is actually part of a money laundering scheme. After reviewing Walker's evidence, Remy is not convinced that illegal activity has occurred, so he consults his firm's legal counsel and shares the client information pointed out by Walker. Did Remy violate the Standard related to client confidentiality?
    A. Remy's actions comply with the Standard.
    B. Consulting with the firm's legal counsel was appropriate, but Remy violated the Standard by sharing client information with Walker.
    C. Sharing client information with Walker was appropriate, but Remy violated the Standard by sharing client information with the firm's legal counsel.

14. Vanessa Richards, CFA, believes MegaRx, a pharmaceutical manufacturer, is likely to require a goodwill writedown in the upcoming year. Richards writes an investment recommendation report with the following statement:

    > "A short strategy is recommended for MegaRx based on the lack of new prescription drugs in the pipeline and the fact that the company will write down goodwill sometime in the near future."

    Richards's supervisor, James Swanson, CFA, reviews the investment recommendation report and approves it for public dissemination. Did Richards or Swanson violate any CFA Institute Standards of Professional Conduct?
    A. No violations by Richards or Swanson occurred.
    B. Richards has violated the Standards, but Swanson has not.
    C. Both Richards and Swanson are in violation of the Standards.

15. A GIPS-compliant firm must:
    A. have its compliance verified by an independent third party.
    B. adjust historical composite returns for relevant changes in firm organization.
    C. provide a compliant performance presentation to every prospective client.

16. With respect to the responsibilities of supervisors, the Code and Standards state that those with supervisory responsibility:
    A. may not delegate supervisory responsibility.
    B. are in violation if an employee under their supervision commits securities fraud.
    C. must institute procedures to prevent and detect violations of rules and regulations by those subject to their supervision.

17. Phillip Kevil, CFA, is an investment advisor for Sensible Investments Inc. One of Kevil's clients, Alan Miller, has requested that Kevil purchase shares of LongShot Technology through a broker that charges higher-than-average fees. Miller maintains a nondiscretionary account and makes each investment decision himself. Even though the account is not discretionary, Miller does allow Kevil to vote all proxies for his account. Kevil generally votes the proxies with management since most of the stocks in Miller's account are high-tech companies in which the managers are the largest shareholders. Has Kevil violated any Standards?
    A. Kevil has not violated any Standards.
    B. Using Miller's choice of broker is not a violation, but Kevil's proxy voting policy is a violation.
    C. Both using Miller's choice of broker and Kevil's proxy voting policy are violations.

18. Gary Hoskins, CFA, runs a macro strategy hedge fund. The hedge fund has a short position in July osmium futures. Hoskins attempts to gain control of the available supply of osmium that can be delivered in July, which will cause holders of long July futures to make offsetting trades instead of settling by delivery. Has Hoskins violated the Standard concerning market manipulation?
    A. Yes.
    B. No, because Hoskins is executing an arbitrage trade.
    C. No, because Hoskins is not manipulating the price of osmium.

Questions 19 through 32 relate to Quantitative Methods. (21 minutes)

19. Tony Borden, CFA, is analyzing the earnings of two companies. For each company, Borden estimates a probability that its earnings will exceed the consensus estimate. To estimate the probability that at least one of the companies will exceed its earnings estimate, Borden should use the:
    A. total probability rule.
    B. addition rule of probability.
    C. multiplication rule of probability.

20. Reinhart Marcs manages a portfolio whose monthly returns follow a distribution with a kurtosis measure of 4.2. Relative to a portfolio with normally distributed returns, Marcs's portfolio has a:
    A. higher chance of extreme upside returns and higher chance of extreme downside returns.
    B. lower chance of extreme upside returns and higher chance of extreme downside returns.
    C. higher chance of extreme upside returns and lower chance of extreme downside returns.

21. For a skewed distribution that has excess kurtosis, the minimum percentage of the distribution within three standard deviations of the mean is *closest* to:
    A. 68%.
    B. 89%.
    C. 99%.

22. Kevin Prince is a technical analyst. Prince has noticed that the price of BHD Corporation has been increasing faster than a broad index of stocks. Prince suggests to his supervisor that BHD stock be added to their clients' portfolios. Prince's recommendation is *most likely* based on which stock price and volume technique?
    A. Divergence.
    B. Moving average.
    C. Relative strength.

23. Which of the following parameters is necessary to estimate the distribution of portfolio returns but not the distributions of individual stock returns?
    A. Mean.
    B. Standard deviation.
    C. Correlation coefficient.

24. A discrete random variable is *best* described as a variable that can be assigned a(n):
A. finite number of possible values.
B. finite number of possible integer values.
C. infinite number of possible integer values.

25. Penny Street, CFA, is considering how to select four stocks out of an industry group of seven to form a weighted portfolio. The portfolio will be weighted 40% to the first stock, 30% to the second stock, 20% to the third stock, and 10% to the fourth stock. The total number of posible weighted portfolios is *closest* to:
A. 35.
B. 168.
C. 840.

26. To determine the value added by active management, a researcher examined the returns of the 20 mutual funds in the large-cap value category that have at least 15 years of returns history available. The results of this analysis *most likely* suffer from:
A. look-ahead bias.
B. time-period bias.
C. survivorship bias.

27. Hugh Benson, CFA, purchases a $100,000 Treasury bill that matures in 90 days for $97,750. If Benson holds the bill until maturity, he will earn a holding period yield (HPY) of 2.3%. To state the return on a different basis, Benson can:
A. multiply the HPY by 365/90 to determine the money market yield.
B. compound the HPY for four periods to calculate the effective annual yield.
C. convert the HPY to a semiannual effective yield and multiply by 2 to calculate the bond equivalent yield.

28. Jane Padgett, CFA, manages a portfolio of low beta stocks for a client. Her client has expressed a strong need to earn a rate of return on the portfolio of at least 4%. The risk-free rate is currently 2%. Which of the following *best* measures the risk Padgett's client is most concerned about?
A. Sharpe ratio.
B. Safety-first ratio.
C. Treynor ratio.

29. Ricky Gould, CFA, is assigned the task of examining the relevance of the capital asset pricing model by running hypothesis tests on the risk-free rate and the market risk premium. Gould forms the following hypotheses:

    Hypothesis 1: For the CAPM to be valid, the mean 1-year Treasury bill rate should equal 4%.

    Hypothesis 2: For the CAPM to be valid, the mean market risk premium should be positive.

    Gould collects historical rate of return data for 1-year Treasury bills and for the annual market risk premium over the past 30 years. To test his hypotheses:
    A. Hypothesis 1 requires a one-tailed test.
    B. Hypothesis 2 requires a one-tailed test.
    C. both Hypothesis 1 and 2 require one-tailed tests.

30. Tiffany Green asks the senior research associate at the Paris Hedge Fund to develop a consistent estimator of the risk associated with the firm's primary hedge fund. Green requires that the estimator:
    A. more accurately estimates the population parameter value as the number of sampled observations increases.
    B. has a variance of sampling distributions less than that of any other estimator.
    C. has an expected value equal to the true population parameter.

31. Sydney Burns, CFA, is considering the purchase of a bond issued by SubPrime Providers. The bond is highly liquid and has a maturity equal to that of a long-term Treasury bond. The SubPrime Providers bond carries a default risk premium of 5%. Burns notices that the difference in interest rates offered on long-term Treasury bonds and short-term Treasury bills currently equals 4%. The real risk-free rate equals 1% and the expected inflation rate equals 2%. Burns should expect the interest rate on the SubPrime Providers bond to:
    A. be greater than or equal to 4%, and less than or equal to 8%.
    B. be greater than or equal to 5%, and less than or equal to 9%.
    C. be greater than or equal to 7%, and less than or equal to 12%.

32. Joe Bay, CFA, wants to test the hypothesis that the variance of returns on energy stocks is equal to the variance of returns on transportation stocks. Bay assumes the samples are independent and the returns are normally distributed. The appropriate test statistic for this hypothesis is a(n):
    A *t*-statistic.
    B. *F*-statistic.
    C. Chi-square statistic.

Questions 33 through 44 relate to Economics. (18 minutes)

33. A manufacturing plant exhibits diseconomies of scale if long-run average cost (LRAC) is:
A. decreasing as output increases, and the plant is at its minimum efficient scale if LRAC is at its lowest level.
B. decreasing as output increases, and the plant is at its minimum efficient scale if LRAC is decreasing over the entire range of output.
C. increasing as output increases, and the plant is at its minimum efficient scale if LRAC is at its lowest level.

34. Consider a market where quantity demanded = 1,500 – 3 × price, and quantity supplied = 2,000 – 5 × price. With respect to equilibrium price and quantity, there is:
A. no market equilibrium.
B. a stable market equilibrium.
C. an unstable market equilibrium.

35. Open market sales of securities by a country's central bank will *most likely* result in:
A. decreasing short-term interest rates.
B. appreciation of the domestic currency.
C. an increasing growth rate of real GDP.

36. If the number of employed and the working age population remain constant, what are the effects of a decrease in the labor force on the unemployment rate and the participation ratio?
A. Both will increase.
B. Both will decrease.
C. One will increase and the other will decrease.

37. Which approach to analysis of trade deficits indicates that in the absence of excess capacity in the economy, currency devaluation provides only a temporary improvement in a country's trade deficit, and that long-term improvement requires either a smaller fiscal deficit or a larger excess of domestic savings over domestic investment?
A. Elasticities approach.
B. Absorption approach.
C. Real wealth approach.

38. With respect to a decrease in the price of a normal good, the income effect:
    A. and substitution effect both tend to increase consumption of the good.
    B. is to decrease consumption of the good, and the substitution effect is to increase consumption of the good.
    C. is to increase consumption of the good, and the substitution effect is to decrease consumption of the good.

39. A consumer's budget constraint is drawn with Good X on the horizontal axis and Good Y on the vertical axis. If the price of Good X decreases from €8 to €6, and the price of Good Y decreases from €20 to €14, the absolute value of the slope of the consumer's budget constraint:
    A. increases.
    B. decreases.
    C. remains the same.

40. Oil Tool Inc. and Jones International Co. are manufacturers in an oligopolistic industry. Oil Tool and Jones enter a covert pricing agreement in which neither will reduce its prices to gain market share. Using the Nash equilibrium model, which outcome is *most likely*?
    A. Both firms will cheat on this agreement.
    B. Neither firm will cheat on this agreement.
    C. Only one of the firms will cheat on this agreement.

41. The national government has undertaken a plan to combat a recession that includes a fiscal stimulus package. The school of economic thought *most likely* to support this action is the:
    A. Neoclassical.
    B. Keynesian.
    C. Monetarist.

42. At a base period, the CPIs of the countries of Tuolumne (currency is the TOL) and Bodee (currency is the BDE) are both 100, and the exchange rate is 0.90 BDE/TOL. One year later, the exchange rate is 0.75 BDE/TOL, and the CPI has risen to 110 in Tuolumne and 105 in Bodee. The real exchange rate is *closest* to:
    A. 0.72 BDE/TOL.
    B. 0.79 BDE/TOL.
    C. 0.83 BDE/TOL.

43. According to the quantity theory of money, the *most* appropriate means to combat inflation is to:
    A. reduce the velocity of money.
    B. reduce the money supply.
    C. increase the excess reserves of banks.

44. The actual incidence of a tax imposed on producers of a good will be borne by:
    A. producers more than consumers if demand for the good is less price elastic than supply.
    B. consumers more than producers if the supply of the good is more price elastic than demand.
    C. consumers and producers equally because the actual incidence of a tax is unaffected by price elasticity.

Questions 45 through 68 relate to Financial Reporting and Analysis. (36 minutes)

45. Information concerning the effects of inflation on a company's operations would *most likely* be found in:
    A. the proxy statement.
    B. the auditor's report.
    C. management's commentary.

46. A classified balance sheet categorizes assets and liabilities based on whether they are:
    A. current or non-current items.
    B. measured at cost or fair value.
    C. internally generated or acquired.

47. Excalibur Equity Fund uses a screen to identify value stocks. Excalibur *most likely* screens for stocks with:
    A. above-average earnings growth rates, which results in an overweighting of technology companies.
    B. below-average price-to-book-value ratios, which results in an overweighting of technology companies.
    C. below-average price-to-book-value ratios, which results in an overweighting of financial services companies.

48. Gus Davy, CFA, is reviewing an industry which has been experiencing rising prices as well as unit volume growth. Davy's investment criteria include selecting companies generating the highest profit margins. If Davy does not adjust companies' financial statements for their inventory cost assumptions, he is *most likely* to select companies that use:
    A. FIFO.
    B. LIFO.
    C. weighted average cost.

49. A company experiences a number of unusual losses during its current fiscal year. Which of these events would *most likely* qualify as extraordinary gains and losses under U.S. GAAP?
    A. Write-down of equipment leased to other companies.
    B. Costs of unexpected damage caused by a plane crash at the company's major plant.
    C. Foreign currency losses from unexpected currency devaluation.

50. At the beginning of the year, BJC Company had 40,000 shares of $1 par common stock outstanding. On April 1, BJC issued a 2-for-1 stock split and on July 1, BJC reacquired 20,000 shares. On October 1, BJC issued 8,000 shares of $10 par, 5% cumulative preferred stock. How many shares should BJC use to calculate diluted earnings per share?
    A. 60,000.
    B. 62,000.
    C. 70,000.

51. A firm's common-size balance sheet shows accounts receivable 5%, inventories 10%, current assets 30%, and current liabilities 25%. Based only on these data, an analyst can determine the firm's:
    A. quick ratio.
    B. defensive interval.
    C. working capital turnover.

52. A company invests $50 million in a bond portfolio yielding 4% with an average maturity of seven years. After one year, interest rates have fallen by 50 basis points. The company will report the highest retained earnings if the securities in the portfolio are classified as:
    A. held-to-maturity.
    B. available-for-sale.
    C. trading securities.

53. Fricks Ltd. is a gold mining company headquartered in Indonesia but with operations throughout the world. Fricks uses International Financial Reporting Standards (IFRS). When subsidiaries located in the United States and Canada pay dividends to the Indonesian parent company, Fricks may classify the dividends as:
    A. cash flow from investing only.
    B. cash flow from financing only.
    C. cash flow from either investing or operations.

54. During 20X3, Shawnee Corp. reported the following transactions:
    - Collected cash from customers totaling $120 million.
    - Paid cash expenses, including taxes, of $96.5 million.
    - Accrued depreciation expense of $6 million.
    - Acquired 30% equity interest in affiliate for $24 million.
    - Collected dividends on stock investments of $3.5 million.
    - Paid a cash dividend of $1.2 million to common shareholders.
    - Sold $4.5 million of treasury stock.

    What amount should Shawnee report as net cash flow from operating activities in its 20X3 cash flow statement according to U.S. GAAP?
    A. $20.0 million.
    B. $23.5 million.
    C. $27.0 million.

55. Vasco Ltd. purchased a unit of heavy equipment one year ago for £500,000 and capitalized it as a long-lived asset. Because demand for equipment of this type has grown significantly, Vasco believes the fair value of its equipment has increased to £600,000. If Vasco revalues its equipment to £600,000, what will be the *most likely* effect on Vasco's financial results, compared to not revaluing the equipment?
    A. Net income will be higher in the period of the revaluation.
    B. The debt-to-equity ratio will be unaffected by the revaluation.
    C. Net income will be lower in the periods following the revaluation.

56. In accordance with U.S. GAAP, JLC Corporation reports its inventory at replacement cost under the lower-of-cost-or-market rule. This implies that the original cost is:
    A. greater than replacement cost, and the net realizable value is less than replacement cost.
    B. greater than replacement cost, and the net realizable value is greater than replacement cost.
    C. less than replacement cost, and the net realizable value is greater than replacement cost.

57. An analyst using vertical common-size analysis is *most likely* to express each item on an income statement as a percentage of:
    A. sales.
    B. operating income.
    C. its value in a base period.

58. At the beginning of the year, Krimp Company evaluated two of the firm's ongoing projects. Krimp's managers judge that a research and development project has completed the research stage and is now in the development stage. They also judge that a software development project has now resulted in a technologically feasible product. Under IFRS, which of these judgments will tend to increase Krimp's income for the year?
    A. Both of these judgments.
    B. Neither of these judgments.
    C. Only one of these judgments.

59. The balance sheet for Jenkins, Inc. is shown below:

Jenkins, Inc. Balance Sheet (In $ millions)

Assets	*20X9*	*20X8*	*Liabilities & Equity*	*20X9*	*20X8*
Current assets			Current Liabilities		
Cash	40	30	Accounts Payable	18	15
Accounts Receivable	8	9	Interest Payable	5	4
Inventory	7	6			
Noncurrent Assets			Noncurrent Liabilities		
Land	40	36	Bonds	23	24
Gross Plant & Equipment	80	82	Deferred Taxes	19	19
Accumulated Depreciation	(17)	(16)	Equity		
Net Plant & Equipment	63	66	Common Stock	41	39
Goodwill	8	12	Retained Earnings	60	58
Total Assets	166	159	Total Liabilities & Equity	166	159

Based on the information in the balance sheet, Jenkins's other financial statements for 20X9 will show a(n):
    A. increase of $4 million on the statement of shareholders' equity.
    B. negative net cash flow of $10 million on the statement of cash flows.
    C. negative cash flow from financing of $2 million related to a repurchase of common stock.

60. Low inventory turnover in a period of declining revenue growth is *most likely* an indication that a firm may have:
    A. obsolete inventory.
    B. too little inventory.
    C. efficient inventory management.

61. Winifred Company's financial statements include the following income tax footnote:

Year	20X5	20X4
Gross deferred tax assets	$133,000	$131,500
Valuation allowance	8,100	11,700

This footnote suggests Winifred's management expects future earnings to:
A. increase.
B. decrease.
C. remain constant.

62. Service costs for a defined benefit pension plan are recognized on the income statement under:
A. IFRS, but not U.S. GAAP.
B. Both IFRS and U.S. GAAP.
C. Neither IFRS nor U.S. GAAP.

63. A firm that chooses the weighted average cost flow assumption for valuing inventory produced by the firm:
A. must use weighted average cost to value all of its inventories.
B. may use first-in-first-out to value similar but distinct inventory items.
C. may use specific identification to value distinguishable high-cost inventory items.

64. U.S. GAAP and IFRS have converged with respect to the treatment of:
A. valuation of inventories.
B. interest received on held-to-maturity securities.
C. unrealized gains on available-for-sale securities.

65. Marquette Industries's return on equity increased from 18% to 21% over the past three years. This increase is *least likely* to be attributed to a(n):
A. increase in Marquette's net profit margin.
B. decrease in Marquette's financial leverage.
C. loss reported in other comprehensive income.

66. A decrease in accumulated depreciation is *most likely* to result from:
A. selling or disposing of a long-lived asset.
B. increasing the salvage value of a long-lived asset.
C. decreasing the estimated useful life of a long-lived asset.

67. JiffyCo's tax rate is 40%. JiffyCo purchases a $200 asset with no salvage value which is depreciated on a straight-line basis for four years for tax purposes and five years for financial reporting. At the end of the second year:
A. JiffyCo's effective tax rate has decresed.
B. the asset's carrying value is greater than its tax base.
C. the deferred tax asset has a balance of $8.

68. Other things equal, what impact will increasing days sales in payables have on operating cash flow?
A. No impact.
B. Lower operating cash flow.
C. Higher operating cash flow.

Questions 69 through 78 relate to Corporate Finance. (15 minutes)

69. To maximize the value of a firm and shareholder wealth, capital projects should be accepted at any point along a firm's investment opportunity schedule that is:
A. above the firm's average cost of capital curve.
B. below the firm's marginal cost of capital curve.
C. above the firm's marginal cost of capital curve.

70. A company's pretax cost of fixed-rate debt capital equals the company's new debt:
A. coupon rate.
B. current yield.
C. yield to maturity.

71. Langler, Inc. is evaluating two capital projects. Langler has a capital budget of $50 million. Project P has an internal rate of return of 24% and a net present value of $5 million. Project Q has an internal rate of return of 18% and a net present value of $12 million. Project P will cost $15 million, and Project Q will cost $48 million. Based on this information, Langler should accept:
A. Project P to earn the higher return on investment.
B. Project Q to maximize shareholder wealth.
C. both projects because they both add value to the firm.

72. If Samor Company's sales increase by 1%, both its earnings before interest and taxes and its earnings per share will increase by 1.5%. This implies that Samor:
A. has fixed operating costs and uses debt financing.
B. uses debt financing but has no fixed operating costs.
C. has fixed operating costs but does not use debt financing.

73. Pierce Motor Company has an operating cycle of 150 days and a cash conversion cycle of 120 days, while Dunhill Motor, Inc. has an operating cycle of 140 days and a cash conversion cycle of 125 days. Based on these figures it is *most likely* that:
A. average days of payables for Dunhill is less than for Pierce.
B. average days of inventory for Dunhill is less than for Pierce.
C. average days of receivables for Dunhill is less than for Pierce.

74. To choose the weights for a firm's weighted average cost of capital (WACC), an analyst should *most* appropriately use the:
A. firm's current debt and equity weights based on market value.
B. firm's stated target capital structure even though recent fund raising has diverged slightly from the target weights.
C. average debt and equity weights based on market value of the firm's competitors.

75. Johnson's Jar Lids is deciding whether to begin producing jars. Johnson's pays a consultant $50,000 for market research that concludes Johnson's sales of jar lids will increase by 5% if it also produces jars. In choosing the cash flows to include when evaluating a project to begin producing jars, Johnson's should:
A. include both the cost of the market research and the effect on the sales of jar lids.
B. include the cost of the market research and exclude the effect on the sales of jar lids.
C. exclude the cost of the market research and include the effect on the sales of jar lids.

76. When computing weighted average cost of capital (WACC), what is the correct treatment of flotation costs, related to raising additional equity capital?
A. Increase the discount rate to account for flotation costs.
B. Adjust the initial project costs by the amount of the flotation costs.
C. Flotation costs are not substantial enough to be considered in adjusting the cost of equity.

77. In early 20X8, a company changed its customer credit terms from 2/10, net 30 to 2/10, net 40. Comparisons of accounts receivable aging schedules at the end of 20X7 and 20X8 are below.

Number of Days	*20X7 $ millions*	*20X8 $ millions*
0–30	380	350
31–60	65	140
61–90	41	35
Over 90	54	55
Total accounts receivable	540	580

The trends in the company's receivables indicate:
A. improved collections on credit accounts.
B. slower payments from credit customers.
C. a higher receivables turnover ratio.

78. Lawrence Clark, CFA, is analyzing GRE Financial's corporate governance policies. Clark notes the following characteristics regarding GRE Financial's corporate governance:

- A majority of GRE Financial's Board is composed of management, which Clark thinks will allow the Board a better understanding of the complicated issues faced by the company.
- There has been considerable speculation about a potential takeover of GRE Financial. GRE's management initiated a poison pill response, defending the action by stating that the speculation was causing key management personnel to leave the company.

Based on the principles of good corporate governance:
A. only the poison pill is in the best interest of shareholders.
B. only the board composition is in the best interest of shareholders.
C. neither the board composition nor the poison pill is in the best interest of shareholders.

Questions 79 through 84 relate to Portfolio Management. (9 minutes)

79. An equally weighted portfolio of five securities has a standard deviation of returns of 10%. The average standard deviation of returns of the five securities is 15%. If another security with a standard deviation of returns of 15% is added to the portfolio, and the weights are adjusted to restore equal weighting, the portfolio's diversification ratio is *most likely* to:
A. increase.
B. decrease.
C. remain unchanged.

80. Which of the following statements about the security market line (SML) is *least accurate*?
    A. The independent variable in the SML equation is the standard deviation of the market portfolio.
    B. The SML measures risk using the standardized covariance of the stock with the market.
    C. Securities plotting above the SML are undervalued.

81. Wayne Johnson is more risk averse than Sandra Colson. If a risk-free asset is not available, Johnson's optimal portfolio will:
    A. be the same as Colson's.
    B. have a lower expected return than Colson's.
    C. have a higher expected return than Colson's.

82. The *least appropriate* factors for a researcher to use in a multi-factor returns generating model are:
    A. statistical factors.
    B. fundamental factors.
    C. macroeconomic factors.

83. The curve representing the set of portfolios that has the highest expected return for a given level of risk is the:
    A. utility curve.
    B. efficient frontier.
    C. indifference curve.

84. An investment manager is *most likely* to be engaging in tactical asset allocation if she:
    A. increases the allocation to tax-free bonds because the investor's effective tax rate has increased.
    B. allocates more than the targeted 10% to emerging market bonds because the sector appears to be undervalued.
    C. allocates 5% to cash, 20% to fixed income, and 75% to equities based on the investor's long time horizon and high risk tolerance.

Questions 85 through 96 relate to Equity Investments. (18 minutes)

85. An investor purchased a stock for $60 a share using margin from his broker. If the initial margin requirement is 40%, and the maintenance margin requirement is 20%, a margin call will initially be triggered below a share price of:
    A. $30.
    B. $45.
    C. $48.

86. A drawback of using the price to book value ratio as a valuation tool is that book value:
A. is not appropriate for valuing firms with primarily financial assets.
B. may not be an accurate indicator of the value of a company's assets and equity.
C. is ineffective in valuing companies that are not expected to continue as going concerns.

87. An industry in which profitability growth is restricted by strong competition among many firms, overinvestment in capacity, and weak brand loyalty is *most likely* in which phase of the industry life cycle?
A. Mature stage.
B. Decline stage.
C. Shakeout stage.

88. Sacco Inc. has nine directors on its board. Board members serve 3-year terms, and three seats are elected annually using a cumulative voting system. If an investor owns 1,000 shares of Sacco common stock, what is the maximum number of votes the investor may cast for one board candidate?
A. 1,000.
B. 3,000.
C. 9,000.

89. An analyst with Guffman Investments has developed a stock selection model based on earnings announcements made by companies with high P/E stocks. The model predicts that investing in companies with P/E ratios twice that of their industry average that make positive earnings announcements will generate significant excess return. If the analyst has consistently made superior risk-adjusted returns using this strategy, which form of the efficient market hypothesis has been violated?
A. Weak form only.
B. Semistrong and strong forms only.
C. Strong, semistrong, and weak forms.

90. Mark King, CFA, is valuing Nacho Inc., a food distributor. Nacho is currently selling for $28 per share and has a 3.0% dividend yield. The risk-free rate is 4%, and the expected return on the market is 8%. King has calculated Nacho's beta to be 1.25. Based on King's analysis, Nacho stock's intrinsic value is $30 per share. King should:
A. invest in Nacho shares.
B. not invest in Nacho shares because the required rate of return is less than the expected rate of return.
C. not invest in Nacho shares because the required rate of return is greater than the expected rate of return.

91. An analyst uses a temporary supernormal growth model to value a common stock. The company paid a $2 dividend last year. The analyst expects dividends to grow at 15% each year for the next three years and then to resume a normal rate of 7% per year indefinitely. The analyst estimates that investors require a 12% return on the stock. The value of this common stock is *closest* to:
    A. $39.
    B. $53.
    C. $65.

92. In a call market:
    A. a single price that clears the market is set periodically.
    B. trades may occur at any time during market hours.
    C. prices are set by the highest dealer bid and the lowest dealer ask price.

93. Creating a bond market index is more difficult than constructing a stock market index due to:
    A. lack of continuous trade data.
    B. little price volatility of bonds.
    C. a less broad universe of bonds versus stocks.

94. Berger Corporation has a profit margin of 10.0%, total asset turnover of 0.75, and a financial leverage ratio of 1.6. Berger's dividend payout ratio is 60%. If these ratios are sustainable for the long term, the best estimate of Berger's growth rate of earnings and dividends is:
    A. 4.8%.
    B. 7.2%.
    C. 7.5%.

95. Increasing which factor in the dividend discount model, without changing the other two, would be *least likely* to increase a stock's price-to-earnings (P/E) ratio?
    A. The expected dividend payout ratio.
    B. The required rate of return on the stock.
    C. The expected constant growth rate of dividends.

96. The primary capital market involves the sale of:
    A. new issues of securities, which are typically distributed by a specialist.
    B. new issues of securities, which are typically distributed by an underwriter.
    C. existing issues of securities, which are typically distributed by an investment bank.

Questions 97 through 110 relate to Fixed Income. (21 minutes)

97. Antun Blasevic, CFA, manages a fixed-income mutual fund which holds a variety of high-yield corporate bonds. His largest position is in Garjun Technologies, which currently trades to yield 8.75%, while the equivalent maturity U.S. Treasury yields only 5.25%. Which of the following is the *most* accurate description of the yield spread between Garjun Technologies and U.S. Treasuries?
A. The yield ratio is 1.67.
B. The absolute yield spread is 67%.
C. The relative yield spread is 350 basis points.

98. A collateralized debt obligation (CDO) *most likely*:
A. is structured with senior and subordinated tranches.
B. consists of a pool of publicly traded securities issued by U.S.-based entities.
C. is sponsored by a financial institution that wants to remove the underlying securities from its balance sheet.

99. Assume that there is a widely accepted belief in the U.S. that 1-year interest rates will remain stable for the foreseenable future. A yield curve derived from spot rates on U.S. Treasury securities shows the following data:

Maturity	Spot Rate
1 year	3.25%
2 years	4.00%
5 years	6.80%
10 years	7.20%

This yield curve is *least* consistent with which theory of the term structure of interest rates?
A. Pure expectations.
B. Liquidity preference.
C. Market segmentation.

100. A 6% U.S. Treasury note is quoted at a price of 97.625 on July 1. The bond pays interest semiannually on March 31 and September 30. On July 1, the clean price of this bond is *closest* to:
A. $946.41.
B. $976.25.
C. $991.17.

101. Yield spreads are *most likely* to widen in a market environment that exhibits:
A. slowing economic growth.
B. high GDP growth rates.
C. lower-than-normal supply of new bond issuance.

102. Samuelson Company has two bond issues outstanding. One is a zero coupon bond. The other has a 10% semiannual coupon. Both bonds have AA credit ratings, 10 years to maturity, and yields to maturity of 7.5%. The zero coupon bond has:
   A. less reinvestment risk and less interest rate risk than the coupon paying bond.
   B. more reinvestment risk and less interest rate risk than the coupon paying bond.
   C. less reinvestment risk and more interest rate risk than the coupon paying bond.

103. In what way is modified convexity different from effective convexity?
   A. Effective convexity takes embedded options into account, while modified convexity does not.
   B. Effective convexity results in a more accurate estimate of a bond's change in price than modified convexity.
   C. Modified convexity can be used with an unequal increase and decrease in yield, while effective convexity can only be used with an equal increase or decrease in yield.

104. Ted Day, CFA, is valuing a callable bond using several scenarios. He is interested in the impact of yield volatility on the value of the bond. If he assumes yield volatility increases, and holds all else constant, the value he estimates for the bond should:
   A. increase.
   B. decrease.
   C. remain the same.

105. Michelle Garcia, CFA, is analyzing two newly issued corporate debt securities for possible purchase by a client. Bond X is a noncallable 10-year coupon bond currently trading at 102.50. Bond Y is a noncallable 10-year coupon bond currently trading at 98.25. Garcia wants to ensure that her client is fully aware of any probable changes in the bonds' values as they approach maturity. Holding interest rates constant, how will each bond's price change as it approaches maturity?
   A. The price of both bonds will decrease.
   B. The price of Bond X will decrease, and the price of Bond Y will increase.
   C. The price of Bond X will increase, and the price of Bond Y will decrease.

106. The bonds of Grinder Corp. trade at a nominal spread of 150 basis points above comparable maturity U.S. Treasury securities. The option adjusted spread (OAS) on the Grinder bonds is 75 basis points. Using this information, and assuming that the Treasury yield curve is flat:
   A. the zero-volatility spread is 75 basis points.
   B. the zero-volatility spread is 225 basis points.
   C. the option cost is 75 basis points.

107. Tony Horn, CFA, is evaluating two bonds. The first bond, issued by Kano Corp., pays a 7.5% annual coupon and is priced to yield 7.0%. The second bond, issued by Samuel Corp., pays a 7.0% annual coupon and is priced to yield 8.0%. Both bonds mature in ten years. If Horn can reinvest the annual coupon payments from either bond at 7.5%, and holds both bonds to maturity, his return will be:
A. greater than 7.0% on the Kano bonds and less than 8.0% on the Samuel bonds.
B. less than 7.0% on the Kano bonds and less than 8.0% on the Samuel bonds.
C. greater than 7.0% on the Kano bonds and greater than 8.0% on the Samuel bonds.

108. Maria Reyes, CFA, recently purchased a 10-year floating rate bond which is reset semiannually. The bond's coupon is based on the 6-month Treasury rate plus 200 basis points with a cap of 8.5%. These floating rate bonds:
A. reach their maximum coupon rate when the 6-month Treasury bill is at 8.5%.
B. have more interest rate risk than comparable floating rate bonds that reset annually.
C. will be priced similar to comparable fixed rate securities if the 6-month Treasury rate has been greater than 7.0% for the past 12 months.

109. Chris Renburg owns the following portfolio of option-free bonds:

Bond	Par value	Market value	Duration
A	$3,000,000	$2,400,000	4.625
B	$3,500,000	$3,600,000	7.322
C	$1,500,000	$1,200,000	9.300
	$8,000,000	$7,200,000	

The duration of Renburg's bond portfolio is *closest* to:
A. 6.6.
B. 6.8.
C. 7.0.

110. Which of the following is *least likely* a characteristic of Treasury Inflation Protected Securities?
A. Coupon rate is the real return.
B. Par value is adjusted for inflation.
C. Coupon rate is adjusted for inflation.

Questions 111 through 116 relate to Derivatives. (9 minutes)

111. A large silver mining corporation is expecting to have large inflows of raw silver resulting from a discovery. The firm expects the first silver inflow to be ready for sale in nine months, followed by the second inflow three months later, and the final inflow three months after that. The mining company is expecting the price of silver to begin a downward trend for the next 15 months and wants to hedge the expected inflows without exposing themselves to credit risk. The *most* appropriate instrument the company should use is a:
A. series of futures contracts expiring in 9, 12, and 15 months.
B. series of forward contracts expiring in 9, 12, and 15 months.
C. swap contract with payments in 9, 12, and 15 months.

112. Derivatives markets are *most likely* to:
A. reduce transactions costs.
B. increase speculation and risk.
C. provide arbitrage opportunities to investors.

113. Pete Morris writes out-of-the-money call options on the stock of Omacon for a premium of $3.00 each. Morris bears the risk of loss only:
A. if the stock price increases above the option strike price.
B. if the stock price decreases below the option strike price.
C. up to the amount of the premium he received.

114. KCE stock is currently selling for $51.13 per share in the market. Six-month American put options on KCE with a strike price of $55 are available, and the risk-free rate of interest is 3.66%. The lower bound for the KCE put options is *closest* to:
A. $2.89.
B. $3.75.
C. $3.87.

115. Mary Hames enters a long FRA with a contract rate of 4.75% and a notional principal of $10 million. The agreement expires in 30 days and is based on 90-day LIBOR. At expiration, 90-day LIBOR is 5.5%. The payoff to Hames at expiration is *closest* to:
A. $12,300.
B. $18,500.
C. $19,000.

116. Frank Holmes, CFA, is reviewing Martha Inc., a distributor. Holmes is interested in the company's European-style call option. Currently, Martha's stock is trading at $33 per share and pays no dividend. The exercise price of both the call and put options is $30, with 80 days to expiration. The current risk-free rate is 5.50%. Martha's put option sells for $2.75. The price of the call option is *closest* to:
A. $3.35.
B. $5.75.
C. $6.10.

Questions 117 through 120 relate to Alternative Investments. (6 minutes)

117. The value of an existing single-family home used for residential purposes will *most likely* be calculated using the:
A. cost approach.
B. income approach.
C. sales comparison approach.

118. An investor who is limited to buying equity shares but is interested in gaining exposure to commodity prices can *best* achieve this exposure by buying:
A. managed futures funds.
B. commodity index exchange traded funds.
C. equities of firms that produce commodities.

119. The effect of survivorship bias on hedge fund risk and returns from historical results is to overstate:
A. both risk and expected returns.
B. expected returns and understate risk.
C. risk and understate expected returns.

120. Which of the following characteristics *most likely* applies to private equity investing?
A. Liquid secondary market.
B. High degree of reliance on manager skill.
C. Relatively short-term investment horizon.

End of Afternoon Session

Exam 1
Morning Session Answers

To get valuable feedback on how your score compares to those of other Level I candidates, use your Username and Password to gain Online Access at schweser.com and choose the left-hand menu item "Practice Exams Vol. 2."

1. A
2. A
3. C
4. C
5. B
6. C
7. A
8. A
9. B
10. C
11. B
12. B
13. B
14. C
15. A
16. B
17. B
18. B
19. C
20. C
21. B
22. A
23. C
24. A
25. C
26. C
27. C
28. C
29. C
30. B
31. B
32. B
33. A
34. B
35. A
36. A
37. C
38. C
39. B
40. B
41. B
42. B
43. C
44. B
45. A
46. A
47. B
48. A
49. B
50. A
51. A
52. C
53. A
54. A
55. C
56. A
57. A
58. C
59. A
60. B
61. B
62. A
63. A
64. B
65. B
66. C
67. A
68. A
69. C
70. A
71. C
72. A
73. B
74. B
75. A
76. B
77. B
78. C
79. A
80. B
81. B
82. A
83. B
84. C
85. A
86. A
87. A
88. C
89. C
90. B
91. A
92. A
93. B
94. A
95. A
96. B
97. C
98. B
99. B
100. C
101. C
102. A
103. C
104. C
105. A
106. A
107. B
108. C
109. C
110. A
111. A
112. B
113. C
114. B
115. C
116. C
117. C
118. B
119. C
120. A

Exam 1
Morning Session Answers

Answers referencing the Standards of Practice address Study Session 1, LOS 1.b, c and 2.a, b, c, except where noted.

1. **A** Both statements are correct. Total firm assets must include fee-paying and non-fee-paying accounts. If a sub-advisor who manages firm assets is selected by the firm, the performance of assets under the sub-advisor's control must be included in the performance of the firm's composite for those assets. (Study Session 1, LOS 4.a)

2. **A** Standard V(C). This Standard requires CFA charterholders and candidates to maintain appropriate records to support investment recommendations. Shredding all of the supporting documents is clearly a violation of the standard. Mason did not violate Standard V(B), however, since she fully described the basic characteristics of the investment. The level of insider buying is not a basic characteristic of an equity security.

3. **C** In accordance with Standard I(B) Independence and Objectivity, Callahan must only issue recommendations that reflect his own independent judgment. If Deininger will not permit him to do so, Callahan must refuse to cover the firm under the conditions specified.

4. **C** Standard VI(C) Disclosure of Conflicts requires members to disclose to their clients any compensation or benefit received by, or paid to, others for the recommendation of services. Sergeant's failure to disclose that he receives legal services for his referral of clients to Chapman is in violation of the Standards.

5. **B** Schultz continued to act in her employer's best interest while still employed and did not engage in any activities that would conflict with this duty until her resignation became effective. Standard IV(A) Loyalty does not prohibit her from contacting clients from her previous firm if she does not get the contact information from the records of her former employer or violate an applicable non-compete agreement.

6. **C** Checking the references given by potential employees is one of the recommended procedures for compliance with Standard I(D) Misconduct. Other recommended procedures are that the firm adopt a code of ethics and inform employees of potential violations and their consequences for disciplinary action. Neither testing employees' knowledge of laws and regulations nor informing them of actual violations by other employees is specified as a recommended procedure.

7. **A** Selling Knoll stock from either the pension fund or Hess's personal account would be trading on material nonpublic information, in violation of Standard II(A) Material Nonpublic Information.

8. **A** While actual knowledge of an upcoming takeover offer is considered material and nonpublic information, the source here, her podiatrist, is not a reliable source so there is no violation of Standard II(A). The information given indicates that Seros has researched the stock and knows it well, so there is no apparent violation of Standard V(A).

9. **B** Misappropriation of client lists is never permitted. Standard IV(A) Loyalty only prohibits solicitation of an old employer's clients prior to ceasing employment with the old firm. It is permissible to take records or files from the old employer if written permission is received.

10. **C** Standard IV(B) Additional Compensation Arrangements requires that members obtain their employer's written consent before accepting any gift or benefit that may create a conflict of interest with their employer. However, in this situation, the gift is coming from a company seeking only to demonstrate their product. Two tickets here are the firm's product, not a lavish gift.

11. **B** In cases where there is a conflict, the appropriate approach is to follow the local regulation, and disclose any conflict in the GIPS-compliant presentation. (Study Session 1, LOS 4.c)

12. **B** Standard I(B) Independence and Objectivity prohibits members and candidates from personally participating in oversubscribed IPOs. The practice is also a violation of Standard VI(B) Priority of Transactions because the personal transaction adversely affects the interests of clients. Accepting the shares is not a violation of Standard VII(A) Conduct as Members and Candidates in the CFA Program because it does not compromise the reputation or integrity of CFA Institute.

13. **B** According to Standard III(C) Suitability, when a member is in an advisory role, he must determine the investor's objectives (risk and return) and constraints, as well as investment experience, and create an Investment Policy Statement (IPS) for his client. Since each investor's constraints and objectives are different, Kent has violated the Standard by not developing an appropriate IPS for Parker. Providing a description of the model is required by Standard V(B) Communication with Clients and Prospective Clients.

14. **C** According to Standard II(B) Market Manipulation, Reynolds is guilty of information-based manipulation by spreading false rumors to induce trading by others.

15. **A** Standard I(C) Misrepresentation does not prohibit members and candidates from providing clients with data on investment products that have guarantees built into their structures. The CDs are in fact guaranteed, and Nicely correctly points out that only the principal is guaranteed.

16. **B** According to Standard III(D) Performance Presentation, members must ensure the accuracy, fairness, and completeness of performance presentations. Standard III(D) prohibits members from implying that future investment returns will reflect past performance.

17. **B** According to Standard II(A) Material Nonpublic Information, there are situations in which a research analyst can be allowed to temporarily move to the investment banking side of the "wall" until all the information is publicly disclosed. Clearly he cannot use any of this information in research, or share it with colleagues.

18. **B** Neither statement is acceptable. Standard VII(B) Reference to CFA Institute, the CFA Designation, and the CFA Program prohibits any claim, such as that in Statement 1, that holding the CFA designation implies the ability to achieve superior results. Statement 2 alters the CFA mark by inserting periods.

19. **C** The random variable in this question has two outcomes: success (earnings increase) or failure (earnings decrease). Any event that produces just one of two possible outcomes is called a Bernoulli trial. The number of successes in a Bernoulli trial is called a binomial random variable. The formula for finding the probability for *x* successes out of *n* trials is:

    Probability for a binomial random variable = ${}_nC_x p^x(1-p)^{(n-x)}$

    where:
    ${}_nC_x$ = the number of combinations of a set of x successes from a total of n trials
    p = the probability of a success in one randomly selected trial (0.75)
    1 – p = the probability of a failure in one randomly selected trial (0.25)

    $${}_8C_5 = \frac{8!}{5!(8-5)!} = \frac{8!}{5!3!} = 56$$

    Probability of five successes out of eight trials = ${}_8C_5(0.75)^5(0.25)^3$ = 56(0.2373)(0.0156) = 0.2073. (Study Session 3, LOS 9.f)

20. **C** Odds for an event equals the ratio of the probability of success to the probability of failure. If the probability of success is 50%, then there are equal probabilities of success and failure, and the odds for success are 1 to 1. (Study Session 2, LOS 8.c)

21. **B** The Sharpe ratio for the large cap fund = 0.083 / 0.43 = 0.193. (The excess return, R_p – RFR, already reflects the risk-free rate.) The Sharpe ratio for the S&P index fund = (0.079 – 0.03) / 0.26 = 0.1885. The large capitalization mutual fund has a higher Sharpe ratio, and hence superior risk-adjusted returns, compared to the S&P 500 index fund. (Study Session 2, LOS 7.i)

22. **A** Tests of the hypothesis that the variance of a normally distributed population is equal to a specific value use a Chi-square test. Hypothesis tests of the equality of the variances of two independent normally distributed populations use an *F*-test. (Study Session 3, LOS 11.i)

23. **C** Tracking error is defined as the difference between the total return on a portfolio and the total return on the index used as a benchmark for the portfolio's performance. (Study Session 3, LOS 9.h)

24. **A** Confidence intervals for a population mean based on a sample are constructed by multiplying the standard error of a point estimate by a reliability factor, and adding this value to, and subtracting it from, the point estimate. Thus, the point estimate is the midpoint of the confidence interval. The probability that the actual value of the parameter is within a confidence interval is the degree of confidence, which equals one minus the degree of significance. Degrees of confidence or significance apply to confidence intervals but not to point estimates. (Study Session 3, LOS 10.h,j)

25. **C** The *p*-value equals the probability that the null hypothesis is true. For instance, the data indicate that there is a 25% probability that the Axxon Industries (population) earnings equal zero, a 4% probability that the Babson Drilling earnings equal zero, and a 1% probability that the Cerex Energy earnings equal zero. The decision rule is to reject the null hypothesis whenever the *p*-value is less than the significance level. Therefore, the null hypothesis should be rejected for Babson Drilling and Cerex Energy, but not for Axxon Industries. (Study Session 3, LOS 11.e)

26. **C** King has designed a trading strategy based on P/E ratios. All the necessary accounting information must be available in order to implement the strategy. At the beginning of a new year, the earnings from the recently ended fiscal year will not be released for several weeks and perhaps months into the new year. By assuming the fiscal year-end earnings are available at the beginning of the new fiscal year, King is introducing a look-ahead bias into her research design. Time period bias refers to a research design in which results are time-specific and cannot be generalized reliably outside the sample period. Data mining bias refers to the likelihood that in repeated testing of data for various strategies or patterns, eventually a pattern will emerge by chance. (Study Session 3, LOS 10.k)

27. **C** $P(AB) = P(A \mid B)P(B) = 0.7 \times 0.8 = 0.56$. The historical data is conditional, where one event affects the probability of another event. (Study Session 2, LOS 8.d,f)

28. **C** Initially, we are told that the probability of randomly selecting an energy company is 15% ("Smith determines that 15% of the stock market universe consists of energy companies"). This is the prior probability. But Smith gathers new information that she can use to update her prior probability—the randomly selected stock recently declared a dividend increase. Intuitively, we know the updated probability will be much higher than 15% because dividend increases are likely to occur much more often for energy companies (90% of the time) than for non-energy companies (30% of the time). Thus, the correct choice must be 35%.

    To obtain the exact answer, we make use of Bayes' formula:

    $$\text{updated probability} = P(E|D) = P(E) \times \frac{P(D|E)}{P(D)},$$

    where:
    - P(E) is the prior probability that the selected company is an energy company.
    - P(D|E) is the probability of the new information (dividend increase) for a given event (energy company).
    - P(D) is the unconditional probability of the new information (dividend increase).

    P(E) is provided in the question as 15%. P(D|E) also is provided in the question as 90%. P(D) is the probability of a dividend increase, which can occur either if the randomly selected company is an energy company or a non-energy company:

    $$P(D) = [P(E) \times P(D|E)] + [P(E^c) \times P(D|E^c)] = [0.15 \times 0.90] + [0.85 \times 0.30] = 0.39.$$

    $$\text{Therefore, updated probability} = 0.15 \times \frac{0.90}{0.39} = 0.346 = 34.6\%$$

    (Study Session 2, LOS 8.n)

29. **C** Nonparametric tests often transform the original data into ranks or signs. The null hypotheses are then stated in terms of ranks or signs. (Study Session 3, LOS 11.j)

30. **B** Using the total probability rule, we can calculate the unconditional probability of an increase in earnings as follows:

$P(H_I) = P(H_I \mid E) \times P(E) + P(H_I \mid E_P) \times P(E_P)$

where:

$P(E) = 0.55$, the unconditional probability of a good economy

$P(E_P) = 0.45$, the unconditional probability of a poor economy

$P(H_I \mid E) = 0.6$, the probability of an increase in HomeBuilder Inc.'s earnings given a good economy

$P(H_I \mid E_P) = 0.3$, the probability of an increase in HomeBuilder Inc.'s earnings given a poor economy

$P(H_I) = 0.60 \times 0.55 + 0.30 \times 0.45 = 0.33 + 0.135 = 0.465 \approx 0.47$. (Study Session 2, LOS 8.h)

31. **B** Mean > median > mode, which means this sample is right skewed. When a sample is right skewed, sample skewness is positive. Because the sample has an even number of observations, we cannot say with certainty that there is an observation equal to the median. Sample kurtosis of 3.0 is the same as the kurtosis of the normal distribution, so excess kurtosis is zero. (Study Session 2, LOS 7.j,k,l)

32. **B** On a financial calculator: PV = –15,000; FV = 0; PMT = 15,000; N=2; CPT→I/Y = 61.8%. (Study Session 2, LOS 6.a)

33. **A** In the short run, a perfectly competitive firm's supply curve is upward sloping, because if the price increases, firms will increase their quantity supplied. The demand curve for a perfectly competitive firm is horizontal. Each firm in a competitive market is a price taker and has no influence on the price of the product. (Study Session 4, LOS 16.c)

34. **B** A decrease in the money supply will cause short-term interest rates to increase, decreasing investment and consumption spending and thereby decreasing AD. A decrease in taxes will increase disposable incomes, consumption spending, and AD. If the foreign exchange value of the domestic currency decreases, the country's products become relatively less expensive to foreign buyers, while foreign goods become relatively more expensive to domestic buyers. As a result, net exports increase, which increases AD. (Study Session 5, LOS 17.h)

35. **A** A reduction in output and increase in price under monopoly decrease consumer surplus and welfare compared to perfect competition. A natural monopoly may have lower costs than several competitive suppliers. Monopolists charge the profit maximizing price, not the "maximum price." (Study Session 4, LOS 16.b)

36. **A** If the minimum wage rate is set above the equilibrium wage rate, it results in excess supply of labor at that wage level and therefore increases unemployment. If the minimum wage is set below the equilibrium wage, then the minimum wage has no effect. (Study Session 4, LOS 13.k)

37. **C** The currency with the higher interest rate should depreciate over time by approximately the amount of the interest rate differential. We know that PKR is expected to appreciate (and thus the VKN depreciate) over the period because the PKR is trading at a forward premium. Thus, VKN should have an interest rate higher than that for PKR by the amount of the forward premium, or approximately 3.0% + 2.3% = 5.3%. (Study Session 6, LOS 21.g)

38. **C** In the Heckscher-Ohlin model, trade results in a redistribution of wealth within each country between workers and the owners of capital. The price of the relatively less scarce (more available) factor of production in each country will increase and cause redistribution of income toward that factor (to workers in a country with a comparative advantage in labor-intensive goods, and to owners of capital in a country with a comparative advantage in capital-intensive goods). The statements describing the Ricardian and Heckscher-Ohlin models are accurate. (Study Session 6, LOS 20.d)

39. **B** The quantity of output at which short-run marginal cost of production is minimized is the same quantity at which the marginal product of inputs (e.g., labor) is maximized. Profit is maximized by producing the output quantity at which marginal revenue equals marginal cost, which is not typically the same quantity at which marginal cost is minimized. The minimum average variable cost is at the output quantity at which it equals marginal cost, but this is also not typically the quantity with minimum marginal cost. (Study Session 4, LOS 15.d)

40. **B** Indirect business taxes are not subtracted because they are included in national income. (Study Session 5, LOS 17.d)

41. **B** In the kinked demand curve oligopoly model, the demand curve facing each firm is more elastic above the current price and less elastic below the current price, because the other firms in the industry will likely match a price decrease by one firm but will not match a price increase.

    The incentive to cheat on price collusion agreements is illustrated by the Prisoner's Dilemma game theory. Price discrimination is the method by which a price seeking firm can increase profits by charging different prices to consumers in distinct groups with differing price elasticity of demand. (Study Session 4, LOS 16.b,d)

42. **B** Even if a supply curve is downward sloping, it still results in a stable equilibrium if it intersects the demand curve from above (i.e., if the supply curve is more steeply sloped than the demand curve). An equilibrium is stable if a price below equilibrium leads to excess demand that will tend to increase the price. An unstable equilibrium results when a downward sloping supply curve intersects the demand curve from below. (Study Session 4, LOS 13.e)

43. **C** Stagflation is a period of economic contraction with increasing inflation, typically brought on by a sharp decrease in aggregate supply. Investments in equities tend to perform poorly in an economic contraction due to decreasing profitability of companies. Fixed income investments decrease in price when nominal interest rates increase due to increases in inflation. Commodity prices tend to increase with inflation. (Study Session 5, LOS 17.k)

44. **B** To reduce inflation, the central bank would attempt to decrease the rate of growth in the money supply. By increasing the interest rate at which member banks may borrow reserves, the central bank can decrease those banks' willingness to lend, which will decrease money supply growth. Open market purchases or a lower reserve ratio would tend to increase money supply growth and inflation. (Study Session 5, LOS 19.h,j)

45. **A** Under the LIFO or weighted average cost inventory valuation methods, perpetual and periodic inventory accounting systems can result in different values for cost of sales, ending inventory, and gross profit. Under FIFO or specific identification, these values are the same for a periodic or perpetual system. (Study Session 9, LOS 29.d)

46. **A** When the company records unbilled or accrued revenue, an asset such as unbilled revenue or accounts receivable is recorded. (Study Session 7, LOS 23.d,f)

47. **B** IFRS does not require three years of comparative financial information. IFRS does not allow the use of extraordinary items. U.S. GAAP permits extraordinary items. (Study Session 7, LOS 24.f)

48. **A** An allowance for uncollectible accounts is a contra asset account to accounts receivable. If this allowance is not present, assets are overstated. The omission of estimated bad debt expense will result in net income being overstated. Liabilities are not affected. (Study Session 8, LOS 25.d)

49. **B** The steps in the financial analysts framework are: (1) State the objective and context of the analysis; (2) Collect data; (3) Process the data; (4) Analyze and interpret the processed data; (5) Report conclusions and recommendations; (6) Update the analysis. In the data processing step, an analyst takes data collected in the previous step and processes it into adjusted financial statements, common-size statements, ratios and graphs, and forecasts. The data collecting step involves taking financial statements, management discussions, and company site visits as inputs and producing organized financial statements and financial data tables. In the analyzing and interpreting step, the analyst uses information collected and processed in the previous steps to answer the questions the analyst posed in the first step of the framework. (Study Session 7, LOS 22.f)

50. **A** Applying the treasury stock method to the warrants, 5,000,000 + [500,000 – (500,000 × \$20) / \$40] = 5,250,000 shares. The options are antidilutive because their exercise price is higher than the average stock price for the year. (Study Session 8, LOS 25.g)

51. **A** The interest coverage ratio is earnings before interest and taxes divided by interest expense. Treating capitalized interest as an expense will increase interest expense while leaving EBIT unchanged. The analyst's adjustment will reduce the interest coverage ratio. (Study Session 9, LOS 30.a)

52. **C** Since equity is 40% of assets, the leverage ratio is 1 / 0.40 = 2.5. Using the traditional DuPont formula, ROE = 8.7% × 2.4 × 2.5 = 52.2%. (Study Session 8, LOS 28.d)

53. **A** Both IFRS and U.S. GAAP allow deferred taxes to be presented as noncurrent on the balance sheet. However, U.S. GAAP classification depends on whether the underlying asset or liability is current or noncurrent. IFRS requires deferred taxes to be presented as noncurrent and under certain circumstances allows them to be netted on the balance sheet. U.S. GAAP requires that deferred taxes be measured using an enacted tax rate, while IFRS allows measurement using an enacted or substantially enacted tax rate. U.S. GAAP does not allow fixed asset revaluation. Deferred taxes resulting from fixed or intangible asset revaluation is recognized in equity under IFRS. (Study Session 9, LOS 31.j)

54. **A** Interest received, dividends received, and interest paid are operating cash flows under U.S. GAAP, and dividends paid are financing cash flows. Interest received and dividends received may be shown as operating or investing cash flows under IFRS. Interest paid and dividends paid may be shown as operating or financing cash flows under IFRS. (Study Session 8, LOS 27.c)

55. **C** CFI includes capital expenditures, the investment in a joint venture, and acquisitions: –100 – 40 – 80 = –220. The dividend from affiliates is included in operating cash flow. CFF is equal to total cash flow minus CFO minus CFI: 340 – 210 – (–220) = 350. (Study Session 8, LOS 27.a)

56. **A** An analyst can use the historical trend in a firm's financial ratios as well as an industry relative comparison to assess the firm's business strategy. A firm producing premium products with a strategy of differentiation should have higher gross margins, higher advertising expenses, and higher research and development expenses relative to firms in its industry that pursue a low-cost-of-production strategy. (Study Session 10, LOS 35.a)

57. **A** The LIFO liquidation causes old inventory to be sold that was accumulated at lower costs, thereby decreasing COGS as a percentage of sales. Lower COGS as a percentage of sales will result in higher gross profit as a percentage of sales. (Study Session 10, LOS 33.d)

58. **C** An allocation of fixed production overhead based on normal production capacity is included in inventory cost. Neither storage costs that are not required as part of the production process nor shipping costs for delivery to the customer are included in inventory cost. (Study Session 9, LOS 29.a)

59. **A** A decrease in the firm's bond rating will increase the required yield on its debt and decrease its market value. A decrease in the market (and book) value of its debt will decrease the firm's reported debt-to-assets ratio (a solvency ratio). A decrease in balance sheet liabilities will increase equity as long as assets are unchanged. (Study Session 9, LOS 32.b and Study Session 15, LOS 53.j)

60. **B** Because the land is valued above its historical cost on the balance sheet, Dubois is using the revaluation model. The land's revaluation up to €2.2 million would have been reflected in shareholders' equity with a revaluation surplus of €200,000. The decrease in fair value to €1.8 million is an impairment below historical cost, which Dubois must recognize. The revaluation surplus will be reduced to zero, and the amount of the writedown below historical cost (€2 million – €1.8 million = €200,000) will be recognized as a loss on Dubois's income statement. This loss, combined with the removal of the revaluation surplus, will decrease shareholders' equity by €400,000. (Study Session 9, LOS 30.g,h)

61. **B** Securitizing accounts receivable increases operating cash flow in the current period. Reducing days' sales in payables (by paying them more promptly) would most likely decrease operating cash flow. Recognizing asset impairments has no effect on the cash flow statement. (Study Session 10, LOS 34.a)

62. **A** 20X9 taxes payable = 0.5 × 5000 = $2,500

20X9 deferred tax asset increase = 0.5 × 200 = $100

20X9 deferred tax liability increase = 0.5 × 600 = $300

adjustment of deferred tax asset = (0.5 / 0.35) × 2000 – 2000 = $857 (increase in tax rate makes DTA more valuable)

adjustment of deferred tax liability = (0.5 / 0.35) × 1000 – 1000 = $429

Income tax expense = taxes payable + ΔDTL – ΔDTA = 2,500 + (300 + 429) – (100 + 857) = $2,272. (Study Session 9, LOS 31.d,e)

63. A The $2 million difference between sales revenue recognized in December and cash collected from these sales is reflected in an accrued revenue account (accounts receivable) on the balance sheet. Unearned revenue results from collecting cash in an earlier period than the goods or services will be delivered (which is when the revenue can be recognized). Unearned revenue is an accrued liability because the company owes goods or services to the buyers. (Study Session 7, LOS 23.d)

64. B The bonds were issued at a premium in 20X5 because the 8% coupon rate exceeded the 6% market interest rate. Since the current market interest rate of 9% is above the coupon rate, Harter can repurchase the bonds at a price below the carrying value. When the carrying value exceeds the reacquisition price, a gain is recognized in the income statement. (Study Session 9, LOS 32.c)

65. B The cash flow to revenue ratio is CFO / revenue, which decreased to 9.0% in 20X9 from 9.6% in 20X8. Note that this ratio is based on cash from operations, not total cash flow.

The decrease in net profit margin (net income / revenue) to 5.8% from 6.6% does not necessarily indicate a decrease in net income because revenue may have increased enough to generate higher income even at the lower profit margin. The negative percentages for plant and equipment represent cash outflows. The company paid cash equal to 8.3% of revenues for plant and equipment during 20X9, a relative increase from 8.0% of revenues in 20X8. (Study Session 8, LOS 27.h,i)

66. C Acquired intangible assets with finite expected useful lives are amortized. Intangible assets with indefinite lives are not amortized but are tested at least annually for impairment. Renewal at a nominal cost means the trademark should be treated as an asset with an indefinite life. (Study Session 9, LOS 30.b)

67. A The quick ratio numerator is cash plus marketable securities plus accounts receivable, and the denominator is current liabilities. The numerator is unaffected by a change in inventory, while the denominator decreases with a decrease in accounts payable, so the quick ratio will increase. (Study Session 8, LOS 28.b)

68. A Components of the change in a net pension asset or liability that are recognized in current period net income under U.S. GAAP are the expected return on plan assets, interest income or expense, and current period service costs. Past service costs and actuarial gains and losses are recognized in other comprehensive income and amortized over time to the income statement. (Study Session 9, LOS 32.k)

69. C To be independent, a board member must not have any material relationship with the firm, its subsidiaries, or its auditors. Holding a significant stock position would align Yu's interests with the interests of the other shareowners. (Study Session 11, LOS 41.c)

70. A A project with an unconventional cash flow pattern (multiple sign changes) can have multiple IRRs or no IRR. Conflicting project rankings between the NPV and IRR methods can occur, but here, the analyst is evaluating a single project. Not enough information is given to determine whether the NPV will be negative, but a single project with a negative NPV will simply be rejected. (Study Session 11, LOS 36.e)

71. C An appropriate short-term investment policy statement should include limitations on the proportions of the total short-term securities portfolio that can be invested in the various types of permitted securities. The policy statement should also include limitations on the types of securities that can be held. It would be overly restrictive, however, to include a specific listing of issuers from which securities could be purchased. (Study Session 11, LOS 40.e)

72. **A** Cash previously spent to perform a feasibility study is a sunk cost which should be ignored. Working capital requirements and cannibalization are factors that should be considered in capital budgeting. (Study Session 11, LOS 36.b)

73. **B** The nominations committee is responsible for reviewing the performance, independence, skills, and experience of board members, as well as for recruiting new board members, creating board nomination policies, and preparing a succession plan for the company's executives. (Study Session 11, LOS 41.e)

74. **B** $\text{Weight}_{debt} = 35 / (35 + 140) = 0.2$

$\text{Weight}_{equity} = 140 / (35 + 140) = 0.8$

After-tax cost of debt = 9%(1 – 0.4) = 5.4%
Cost of equity = 4% + 0.9(4.5%) = 8.05%
WACC = 0.2(5.4%) + 0.8(8.05%) = 7.52%

(Study Session 11, LOS 37.a)

75. **A** Both statements are accurate. The marginal cost of capital reflects the average risk of a firm's activities and must be adjusted to evaluate projects that are more or less risky than average. Using the marginal cost of capital implicitly assumes that the capital structure of the firm will remain at the target capital structure over the life of the project. (Study Session 11, LOS 37.e)

76. **B** Longer operating and cash conversion cycles are frequently signs of liquidity problems. Slower collections or inventory turnover lengthen the operating cycle. The cash conversion cycle is also growing longer, which suggests the company is not stretching payables to offset the lengthening operating cycle. (Study Session 11, LOS 40.c)

77. **B** Using the constant growth dividend model, the price for a common stock is:

$$P_0 = \frac{D_1}{k_{ce} - g}$$

Solving for k_{ce}:

$$k_{ce} = \frac{D_1}{P_0} + g$$

where:
P_0 = current stock price
D_1 = year end expected dividend
k_{ce} = cost of common equity capital
g = sustainable (constant) growth of equity, earnings, and dividends

The sustainable growth for a company's dividends equal the ROE times the earnings retention rate. The earnings retention rate equals 1 minus the dividend payout rate. Therefore:

$g = 0.15 \times (1 - 0.20) = 0.12$

$$k_{ce} = \frac{D_1}{P_0} + g = 0.05 + 0.12 = 0.17 = 17\%$$

(Study Session 11, LOS 37.h)

78. **C** Given that the NPV is negative, the discount rate used by the company evaluating the project must be greater than the IRR (the discount rate for which the NPV equals zero). On a financial calculator: CF0 = –2.5; CFj = 1; Nj = 3; CPT IRR = 9.7%. Since the discount rate used for this project is greater than 9.7%, it must be closer to 10% than to either of the other answer choices. (Study Session 11, LOS 36.d)

79. **A** Both stocks have the same total risk, but Shaw has more systematic risk (higher beta) than Melon. In equilibrium, both stocks will plot on the Security Market Line, and the expected return will be greater for the higher-beta stock. (Study Session 12, LOS 44.c,f,h)

80. **B** Steeper indifference curves indicate greater risk aversion. Individuals with steeper indifference curves will choose optimal portfolios with lower levels of risk than an individual with a less steep indifference curve. The optimal portfolio for an investor occurs at the point of tangency between the investor's highest attainable indifference curve and the Markowitz efficient frontier. Since individuals have differing levels of risk aversion, they will have different points of tangency and different optimal portfolios. (Study Session 12, LOS 43.d)

81. **B** The standard deviation for a combination of a risky asset, A, and a risk-free asset, F, equals $w_A\sigma_A$ because the standard deviation of a risk-free asset, by definition, is zero. So, Hull's standard deviation equals 0.40(0.20) = 8%. (Study Session 12, LOS 44.a)

82. **A** Endowments and foundations invest for the long term to provide ongoing funding for a specific purpose or charitable cause. They typically have relatively low cash payout rates as a percentage of total assets. Their investment needs are best characterized as long time horizons, low liquidity needs, and high risk tolerance. (Study Session 12, LOS 42.b)

83. **B** When taken together, the asset classes should approximate the investor's total investible universe. Properly defined and specified asset classes should each have a low return correlation to the other asset classes, and within each asset class should be assets that have similar expected risk and return. (Study Session 12, LOS 45.f)

84. **C** The standard deviation of return of a portfolio of many risky assets can be less than or greater than the standard deviation of the least risky asset, depending on the correlations of returns among the assets and their weights in the portfolio. However, the portfolio standard deviation must be less than or equal to the standard deviation of the most risky asset. (Study Session 12, LOS 43.e)

85. **A** An important reason for secondary markets is to provide liquidity to investors after securities are issued. Financial futures are traded on secondary markets. Private placements are not traded, but issued directly to an investor. (Study Session 13, LOS 46.b,i)

86. **A** Because the S&P 500 index is market capitalization weighted, stocks with higher market capitalization have greater influence on the performance of the index. Because the index outperformed its equally weighted version, larger capitalization stocks performed better than smaller capitalization stocks. (Study Session 13, LOS 47.d,e,k)

87. A $RFR_{nominal} = (1 + RFR_{real})(1 + IP) - 1 = (1.04)(1.05) - 1 = 1.0920 - 1 = 0.0920 =$ 9.20%

Using the CAPM, the required rate of return $(k_e) = RFR_{nominal} + \beta(R_{mkt} - RFR_{nominal})$ $= 9.20\% + 1.4(14.0\% - 9.2\%) = 9.20\% + 6.72\% = 15.92\%$

The retention ratio (RR) = 1 – dividend payout ratio = 1 – 0.30 = 0.70

The growth rate $(g_c) = (RR)(ROE) = (0.70)(10\%) = 7.00\%$

$D_0 = E_0(\text{dividend payout}) = \$4.00(0.30) = \$1.20$

Next year's dividend $(D_1) = D_0(1 + g_c) = \$1.20(1 + 0.07) = 1.284$

$P_0 = D_1 / (k_e - g) = 1.284 / (0.1592 - 0.07) = 14.39$

(Study Session 14, LOS 51.h)

88. C The value of preferred stock is the preferred dividend divided by the required rate of return on the preferred. Earnings growth rates do not factor into the valuation of preferred stock since the dividend is typically fixed. Therefore, neither a historical price-to-earnings model nor a multistage dividend discount model is appropriate. (Study Session 14, LOS 51.d)

89. C An alternative trading system that does not reveal current client orders is referred to as a dark pool. Dark pools provide traders anonymity by not revealing their orders to potential counterparties. (Study Session 13, LOS 46.d)

90. B Because the after-tax cost of debt is typically less the than the earnings yield on the stock, issuing debt and repurchasing common stock is most likely to increase ROE, although the variability of net income will be increased (increased financial leverage). Changes in the market value of the common stock will not affect ROE. (Study Session 14, LOS 49.h)

91. A Fundamental analysis (i.e., analysis of public non-market data) can produce positive risk-adjusted returns if markets are weak-form efficient but not semistrong-form efficient. Under the semistrong form of the EMH, fundamental analysis cannot consistently achieve positive risk-adjusted returns. (Study Session 13, LOS 48.e)

92. A Investors are less likely to participate in markets when they believe are at a disadvantage to more informed traders (insiders). By enforcing regulations that prohibit insider trading, a market should attract a larger number of participants and, therefore, increase market efficiency on balance. (Study Session 13, LOS 46.l, 48.c)

93. B Since Marvin is given the real risk-free rate and nominal growth in net income, he will need the inflation rate to either state all inputs on a nominal or real basis. Marvin will also need the expected long-term earnings retention rate to estimate the long-term growth rate for the company. (Study Session 14, LOS 51.c,e)

94. A In a sponsored DR, voting rights of the shares are held by the investor. In an unsponsored DR, voting rights are retained by the depository bank. An advantage of DR shares over direct investments in foreign companies is that DR shares trade in the investor's domestic market and currency. (Study Session 14, LOS 49.d)

95. **A**

	Delmar	*Bell United*
Stock price per share	\$25	\$35
Cash flow = NI + depreciation	\$100 + 250 = 350	\$1,500 + 800 = 2,300
Cash flow per share	350 / 100 = 3.5	2,300 / 500 = 4.6
Price to cash flow ratio	25 / 3.5 = 7.14×	35 / 4.6 = 7.61×

The price/CF multiple indicates that Delmar is a less expensive stock. (Study Session 14, LOS 51.h)

96. **B** Defensive stocks (with low betas and low systematic risk) are less sensitive to economic cycles. A high beta stock is a cyclical stock. Stocks with low P/E ratios are value stocks. (Study Session 14, LOS 50.c)

97. **C** The duration of the Dewey bonds = – (percentage change in price) / (change in yield in percentage points) = – (–4.0) / 0.50 = + 8.0. Dollar duration = duration / 100 × portfolio value = 8 / 100 × \$12 million = \$960,000. (Study Session 15, LOS 53.f)

98. **B** A bond issued at a yield higher than its coupon will be priced below par, or at a discount. Three months later, the yield has declined to 4.2% and the bond will trade at a premium to par, reflecting the fact that the coupon is now higher than the yield. (Study Session 15, LOS 53.b)

99. **B** The advisor's description of the sources of return from investing in a bond is incomplete because it does not include the income from reinvesting the bond's coupon payments. An investor will realize a capital gain or loss at maturity if the bond was priced at a discount or premium when the investor bought it. (Study Session 16, LOS 57.a)

100. **C** $$\left(\frac{(1.035)^4}{(1.025)^2}\right)^{\frac{1}{2}} - 1 = 4.51\%$$

Alternatively, (4 × 3.5 – 2 × 2.5) / 2 = 4.5%. (Study Session 16, LOS 57.g)

101. **C** You can answer this question without calculations. A decrease in interest rates must cause the price to increase. Because duration alone will underestimate a price increase, the price must increase by more than 10%.

percentage change in price = [duration × Δy] + [convexity × (Δy)^2] × 100

decrease in rates = {[10 × 0.01] + [200 × (0.01)^2]} × 100 = 12%

(Study Session 16, LOS 58.h)

102. **A** For bonds with the same credit rating, default rates for municipal bonds have been lower than those of corporate bonds. (Study Session 16, LOS 59.j)

103. **C** Since this is a one-time expenditure, the MTN format with debt issued repeatedly on a best-efforts basis would not be particularly appropriate. The secured bonds would be lower risk for investors than debentures (which are unsecured) and so would probably have the lowest yield. (Study Session 15, LOS 54.h)

104. **C** The duration of a bond can be estimated using the following equation:

$$\frac{\text{Price if yields decline} - \text{price if yields rise}}{2 \times (\text{initial price}) \times (\text{change in yield in decimal})} = \frac{107.42 - 101.38}{2 \times 104.50 \times 0.0025} = 11.56$$

(Study Session 16, LOS 58.e)

105. **A** To value the bond using spot rates, add the zero-volatility spread of 1.5% (150 bp) to each Treasury spot rate and discount the bond's cash flows using these rates. The price of the bond is $5 / 1.05 + 105 / 1.055^2 = 99.10$. (Study Session 16, 57.e,f)

106. **A** The price of a putable bond equals the price of an otherwise identical, yet non-putable, bond plus the price of the bond put option. The price of the bond put option increases when interest rate volatility increases. Therefore, the price of the putable bond will rise. The price of a callable bond equals the price of an otherwise identical, yet non-callable, bond minus the price of the bond call option. The price of the bond call option increases when interest rate volatility increases. Therefore, the price of the callable bond will fall. The price of a floating rate bond will not change significantly, especially if the coupon reset dates are not far apart. (Study Session 15, LOS 53.n)

107. **B** Bond X = 1000 / 950 = 1.0526; Bond Y = 1000 / 850 = 1.1765

80 / (1.0526) = 76; 1080 / (1.1765) = 917.98

Bond Z = 76 + 917.98 = 993.98 ≈ 995

The arbitrage-free valuation approach applies time appropriate spot interest rates to each cash flow of the bond. (Study Session 16, LOS 56.f)

108. **C** Bond Z has no provisions for early retirement (which favor the issuer), so it should yield the lowest. Bond X is noncallable, but allows the issuer to redeem principal through an accelerated sinking fund. Bond Y has an accelerated sinking fund and is callable, giving the issuer the most options, and therefore requiring the highest yield. (Study Session 15, LOS 52.d,e)

109. **C** On-the-run Treasury securities are the most recently auctioned issues. After they are auctioned in the primary market, on-the-run Treasury securities trade in the secondary market alongside off-the-run Treasury securities. On-the-run issues are generally the most actively traded Treasury securities. (Study Session 15, LOS 54.b,k)

110. **A** A bond trading at a discount will have a YTM greater than its coupon. The current yield is 8 / 97.55 = 8.2%. Know the terminology: nominal yield = coupon rate. (Study Session 16, LOS 57.b)

111. **A** For JonesCorp as the fixed-rate receiver (i.e., the floating-rate payer) to make a net payment, LIBOR must increase above the swap fixed rate. Since LIBOR is currently equal to the fixed rate on the swap, the LIBOR term structure would need to either remain flat but shift up or become upward sloping. In either of these scenarios, future LIBOR will be higher than the fixed rate on the swap and JonesCorp will owe more to the counter party than it will receive. (Study Session 17, LOS 64.b)

112. **B** Profit on underlying stock = \$27.13 – \$25.96 = \$1.17
Profit on put option = $\text{Max}(0, X - S_T) - p_0$ = 0 – \$0.65 = –\$0.65
Profit on protective put position = \$1.17 – \$0.65 = \$0.52

(Study Session 17, LOS 65.b)

113. **C** Since Black is hedging part of its production, the company will be short futures. To close out the position, Black would offset the position with a long position on the same exchange. (Study Session 17, LOS 62.e)

114. **B** The minimum value of a European put is Max{0, $[X / (1 + RFR)^T] - S$}, where *X* is the strike price, *S* is the price of the underlying stock, and *T* is the time to expiration. The minimum value of an in-the-money American put is Max[0, (X – S)]. Because the present value of *X* must be less than *X*, the theoretical minimum value of a European put is less than the theoretical minimum value of an equivalent American put. (Study Session 17, LOS 63.j)

115. **C** For a long call position, the profit is equal to the value of the call at expiration minus the initial cost of the call. If the call expires in the money, the value is equal to the final stock price minus the exercise price. Since the final stock price has no upper limit (i.e., it can rise infinitely), the expiration value of the call (and thus the profit) is unlimited. Since the current market price of ZXC ($33.75) is greater than the strike price of the call options ($30), the options are in the money (i.e., they would have value if exercised today). Breakeven occurs when the stock price is equal to the exercise price plus the cost of the option. For ZXC stock, the breakeven stock price is $34.50, not $38.25. (Study Session 17, LOS 65.a)

116. **C** When an investor establishes a futures position, he must deposit initial margin, which is determined by the exchange. As the value of the underlying asset (and thus the futures contract) changes, the balance in the margin account will also change as the account gets marked to market. If the balance falls below the maintenance margin, then the investor will need to deposit additional funds in order to bring the margin account balance back to the initial margin level. The amount required to bring the balance back to the initial level is known as the variation margin. Kent incorrectly reversed the definitions of maintenance and variation margin. Ramsey's statement about the daily settlement price is correct. (Study Session 17, LOS 62.c)

117. **C** Contango refers to the situation where futures prices are greater the spot price, while backwardation refers to the situation where futures prices are less than the spot price. No special name is given to the condition when spot and futures prices are equal. (Study Session 18, LOS 67.a)

118. **B** With a soft hurdle rate, the incentive fee is a percentage of the entire return once the hurdle rate is met. With a hard hurdle rate, the incentive fee is a percentage of return in excess of the hurdle rate. A high water mark does not affect the incentive fee for an account that has increased in value each period. A soft hurdle rate would result in incentive fees of 20% × 8% = 1.6% of assets; a 5% hard hurdle rate would result in incentive fees of 20% × (8% – 5%) = 0.6% of assets; and a 7% hard hurdle rate would result in incentive fees of 20% × (8% – 7%) = 0.2% of assets. (Study Session 18, LOS 66.f)

119. **C** When valuing real estate by comparable sales, an analyst should observe the prices from recent transactions for other similar (comparable) properties and adjust for the specific characteristics of the property being valued. Discounting future cash flows from a real estate property is the income approach. (Study Session 18, LOS 66.e)

120. **A** In a management buy-in, a leveraged buyout (LBO) fund replaces the existing managers of a portfolio company with a new team it believes can increase the value of the company. Companies with high cash flow are attractive candidates for LBOs because their cash flow can help service the debt issued to finance the LBO. A company with high cash flow and capable managers is a potential candidate for a management buyout (MBO), a transaction in which the managers participate and stay on after the company goes private. (Study Session 18, LOS 66.d)

Exam 1
Afternoon Session Answers

To get valuable feedback on how your score compares to those of other Level I candidates, use your Username and Password to gain Online Access at schweser.com and choose the left-hand menu item "Practice Exams Vol. 2."

1. A	31. B	61. B	91. A
2. C	32. C	62. B	92. B
3. B	33. B	63. C	93. B
4. A	34. A	64. C	94. B
5. A	35. C	65. C	95. B
6. B	36. B	66. B	96. C
7. A	37. C	67. B	97. C
8. A	38. B	68. C	98. C
9. B	39. C	69. B	99. B
10. A	40. B	70. C	100. C
11. B	41. A	71. A	101. A
12. B	42. A	72. C	102. C
13. A	43. C	73. B	103. B
14. A	44. B	74. C	104. A
15. A	45. C	75. B	105. C
16. C	46. C	76. C	106. B
17. A	47. C	77. C	107. B
18. A	48. A	78. B	108. B
19. C	49. B	79. C	109. C
20. A	50. B	80. A	110. C
21. C	51. B	81. C	111. B
22. A	52. C	82. B	112. B
23. C	53 A	83. A	113. A
24. B	54. A	84. C	114. B
25. A	55. B	85. A	115. C
26. A	56. B	86. B	116. B
27. C	57. C	87. A	117. A
28. A	58. C	88. B	118. A
29. C	59. B	89. A	119. B
30. C	60. A	90. A	120. B

Exam 1
Afternoon Session Answers

Answers referencing the Standards of Practice address Study Session 1, LOS 1.b, c and 2.a, b, c, except where noted.

1. **A** Under Standard I(C) Misrepresentation, members and candidates may employ ideas from others with proper acknowledgement. By reviewing the third-party research before distributing it, Laird complies with Standard V(A) Diligence and Reasonable Basis. Standard I(B) Independence and Objectivity concerns outside parties who may wish to influence an analyst's independent judgment.

2. **C** Under GIPS, a composite must include all fee-paying discretionary portfolios managed with the same objective or strategy. This standard is designed to prevent firms from selectively including well-performing portfolios in composites. Only discretionary fee-paying portfolios (not all discretionary portfolios) must be included in a composite. (Study Session 1, LOS 4.a)

3. **B** In accordance with Standard VI(B) Priority of Transactions, employer and client transactions must take priority over any personal transactions, meaning any transactions in which the member or candidate is the beneficial owner. Disclosure is not enough; in this instance the personal transaction would take priority over the clients' transactions, which is a violation. "May purchase Maxima at any time, as long as the execution price is not more favorable than the execution price given to the clients" is incorrect because Jones could be purchasing the stock ahead of clients, which is not permitted.

4. **A** Under the mosaic theory, financial analysts are free to combine public information with nonmaterial nonpublic information and act based on their conclusions. Standard II(A) prohibits members and candidates from acting or causing others to act on material nonpublic information. The obligation to make the reasonable efforts to achieve public dissemination of nonpublic information applies to situations in which the company discloses information to the analyst that has not yet been made public.

5. **A** Because the gift depends on Tegger's future performance, Standard IV(B) Additional Compensation Arrangements requires Tegger to obtain permission from his employer before accepting it. This allows the employer to determine whether other accounts may be disadvantaged.

6. **B** Recommended procedures to comply with Standard III(B) Fair Dealing state that initial recommendations should be made available to clients who have indicated an interest in the specific security type. The firm does not need to communicate a recommendation to all clients, but choosing which clients receive the recommendation should be based on suitability and known interest. Differentiated levels of service are acceptable, but not if any client group is disadvantaged. Delaying the distribution of a new or changed recommendation to clients who have expressed an interest would disadvantage them.

7. **A** Since the information that the fund intends to sell shares is nonpublic and is also material (an investor considering sale or purchase of the shares would want to know it prior to making a decision), Rice is prohibited from acting on it by Standard II(A) Material Nonpublic Information. Rice has also violated Standard VI(B) Priority of Transactions by not executing the client sell order prior to selling his own shares.

8. **A** GIPS are understandably not all-inclusive, and firms are encouraged to include supplemental firm-specific information within the GIPS-compliant presentation of investment results. (Study Session 1, LOS 4.d)

9. **B** Standard IV(C) Responsibilities of Supervisors requires members to make a reasonable effort to prevent their subordinates from violating laws, regulations, rules, and the Code and Standards, and to identify such violations. A member should decline supervisory responsibility in writing if proper compliance procedures are not in place.

10. **A** GIPS are voluntary standards. If an investment firm chooses to follow and comply with GIPS, GIPS-compliant investment performance results must be adhered to for both existing and prospective clients. (Study Session 1, LOS 3.a)

11. **B** A complete withdrawal from market-making activities could be a signal to outsiders that a significant transaction is underway. The firm should continue making a market but should only carry out unsolicited transactions for clients.

12. **B** Under Standard VI(C) Referral Fees, Pollard is required to inform his clients and his employer of the arrangement with Timberlake. Disclosure allows the employer and clients to evaluate any possible partiality shown in the direction of trades and also the full cost of the services. Standard I(B) Independence and Objectivity is intended to apply to situations in which the member may face pressure to recommend investments or take investment action contrary to his independent judgment.

13. **A** Standard III(E) Preservation of Confidentiality applies to the confidential information of both current and former clients of the member or candidate. The Professional Conduct Program is considered an extension of the member or candidate with respect to preservation of confidentiality. The Standard does not prohibit the member or candidate from disclosing confidential information to authorities that concerns illegal activity.

14. **A** Standard I(B) Independence and Objectivity requires that analyst recommendations must reflect their own objective views. Analysts must not yield to pressure from other departments. Any action by Lear to influence the analysts' recommendations as Hall requested would violate this Standard. Lear's most appropriate action is to have the firm's compliance department place Versoxy on the restricted list, and only offer factual information (rather than a recommendation) about the company to clients while the stock offering is in progress.

15. **A** The GIPS-compliant firm definition must be the corporation, subsidiary, or division that holds itself out to the client as a specific business entity. If the firm has different geographic locations, this firm definition should include all the locations. (Study Session 1, LOS 4.b)

16. **C** Todd may not claim that she is a "Level III candidate in the CFA program" because she has not registered for the next Level III CFA examination. There is no partial designation for someone who has passed Level I, Level II, or Level III of the CFA examination.

17. A Because Anderson is an independent contractor, rather than an employee of U.S. Securities, Anderson only needs to abide by the terms of his agreement with U.S. Securities to be in compliance with Standard IV(A) Loyalty.

18. A Standard I(D) Misconduct prohibits members from participating in any professional conduct that reflects adversely on their professional reputation or integrity. Declaring personal bankruptcy does not, by itself, reflect adversely on the individual's integrity or trustworthiness. If the circumstances of the bankruptcy included any fraudulent or deceitful conduct on the part of the member, then that would be considered a violation.

19. C First, Mann created 10 firm size groups (deciles). Then, within each of the 10 deciles, he created 5 P/E groups (quintiles), for a total of 50 classifications. (Study Session 2, LOS 7.f)

20. A Because the distribution is continuous, the probability of any specific outcome is zero. (Study Session 3, LOS 9.i)

21. C The chi-square test is sensitive to violations of its assumptions. If the population from which the sample is drawn is not normally distributed, then inferences based on the chi-square test will be flawed. (Study Session 3, LOS 11.i)

22. A Both statements are considered to be advantages of technical analysis. (Study Session 3, LOS 12.a)

23. C $\sigma_p = \sqrt{w_1^2\sigma_1^2 + w_2^2\sigma_2^2 + 2w_1w_2\sigma_1\sigma_2\rho_{1,2}}$

Given $\rho_{1,2} = +1$, $\sigma_p = \sqrt{(0.5)^2(0.1)^2 + (0.5)^2(0.3)^2 + 2(0.5)(0.5)(0.1)(0.3)} = 20\%$

Note also that with $\rho_{1,2} = 1$, the portfolio standard deviation is a weighted average of the asset standard deviations, 0.5(10) + 0.5(30) = 20%. (Study Session 2, LOS 8.l)

24. B Time-series data refer to observations spread out over time for one entity (company, fund, etc.). In contrast, cross-sectional data refer to observations spread out over many entities but measured over one period of time. McWyllie examines the relationship between price-to-equity and debt-to-equity ratios for many companies, over a single period of time. He uses data representing a broad cross-section of the U.K. market, over a specific period of time. (Study Session 3, LOS 10.d)

25. A A positive NPV project will have an IRR greater than the WACC, while a negative NPV project will have an IRR less than the WACC. The NPV method assumes reinvestment at the opportunity cost of capital (i.e., the weighted average cost of capital). NPV measures the additional shareholder wealth created by an investment project. A project with zero NPV will increase the size of the firm but will not add to shareholder wealth. (Study Session 2, LOS 6.b)

26. A Shortfall risk refers to the probability that the investment will fail to earn a pre-specified minimum acceptable (threshold) return. Jackson's pension portfolio threshold return equals 7%. Notice that the threshold return is 2 standard deviations below the portfolio expected return:

$$z = \frac{0.07 - 0.15}{0.04} = -2.0$$

Using the normal probability distribution, the probability that z will be less than −2 is approximately 2.5%. (Study Session 3, LOS 9.m,n)

27. C coefficient of variation $= \dfrac{\text{standard deviation}}{\text{mean return}}$

sharpe ratio $= \dfrac{\text{asset return} - \text{risk-free rate}}{\text{standard deviation}}$

	Coefficient of Variation	Sharpe Ratio
Real Estate	0.18 / 0.25 = 0.72	(0.25 – 0.04) / 0.18 = 1.17
Fixed Income	0.04 / 0.08 = 0.50	(0.08 – 0.04) / 0.04 = 1.00
Equities	0.15 / 0.20 = 0.75	(0.20 – 0.04) / 0.15 = 1.07

(Study Session 2, LOS 7.i)

28. A The probability of high momentum (M) is conditional on the stock being among the small cap stocks (S). The conditional probability of finding a high earnings momentum stock given that the stock is small is expressed as:

$P(M \mid S) = 0.40$

To satisfy Murphy's criteria, a stock must be a small-cap stock and have high earnings momentum. The joint probability is calculated as the product of the conditional probability and the unconditional probability of being a small-cap stock:

$P(M \text{ and } S) = P(M \mid S)\, P(S) = 0.40 \times 0.20 = 8\%$ (Study Session 2, LOS 8.f)

29. C The hypothesis test is a two-tailed test of equality of the population means. The *t*-statistic is greater than the critical *t*-value. Therefore, Ratliff can reject the null hypothesis that the population means are equal. (Study Session 3, LOS 11.g)

30. C Stratified sampling divides the population according to common characteristics and then selects samples from each subgroup in proportion to the subgroup's representation in the overall population. (Study Session 3, LOS 10.c)

31. B A histogram is a bar chart representing the relative frequencies of observations in the sample (i.e., the frequency distribution). (Study Session 2, LOS 7.d)

32. C Because the sample size is large (typically defined as a sample size greater than 30), we can use the normal probability approximation to answer this question. We can either use the normal probability table (or simply recall from memory) that the appropriate critical value associated with the 90% confidence interval (using the normal probability distribution) is 1.645. Therefore, using the sample data provided in the question, the 90% confidence interval for the population mean is approximately:

sample average ± 1.65(Standard Error)

The standard error equals the sample standard deviation divided by the square root of the sample size:

$$\text{standard error} = \frac{\$50{,}000{,}000}{\sqrt{100}} = \frac{\$50{,}000{,}000}{10} = \$5{,}000{,}000.$$

Therefore, using the large sample approximation, the 90% confidence interval for the population mean equals:

\$2 million ± 1.65(\$5 million) = \$2 million ± \$8.25 million = –\$6.25 million to \$10.25 million.

(Study Session 3, LOS 10.j)

33. B At interest rates below 4% (the long-term equilibrium rate), the quantity of money demanded exceeds the quantity of money supplied. At below-equilibrium rates, investors will sell bonds to obtain the desired extra cash. As they sell more bonds, the prices of bonds fall, and interest rates start to move back towards the 4% equilibrium. (Study Session 5, LOS 19.d)

34. A Open market operations to sell securities will decrease the outstanding supply of cash balances and increase short-term interest rates. The central bank does not issue long-term bonds but may buy and sell bonds issued by the government. Decreasing reserve requirements or purchasing government securities would tend to decrease short-term interest rates. (Study Session 5, LOS 19.h and Study Session 15, LOS 55.a)

35. C Under a currency board arrangement, the monetary authority agrees to exchange its domestic currency for a foreign currency at a fixed rate. A fixed peg arrangement allows variation within a band of ±1% around the target exchange rate. With dollarization, a member country does not have a domestic currency of its own. (Study Session 6, LOS 21.h)

36. B Successful collusion is unlikely in a market that can be characterized as monopolistic competition because low entry barriers would allow new competitors to emerge. Firms in such an industry can earn short-run economic profits and often differentiate their products on quality or price. (Study Session 4, LOS 16.a,b)

37. C Frictional unemployment results from the time necessary to match workers with available jobs and is not related to economic cycles. Cyclical unemployment results from economic cycles. Singh's description of structural unemployment is accurate. (Study Session 5, LOS 18.d)

38. B Since the Munich plant is generating revenues greater than costs and the Paris plant is not, Hanover should increase output at the Munich plant and reduce output at the Paris plant. (Study Session 4, LOS 15.g)

39. **C** The cross elasticity of demand for goods that are complements is negative because an increase in the price of one would tend to decrease the quantity demanded of the other. The cross elasticity of demand for substitute goods is positive because an increase in the price of one would tend to increase the quantity demanded of the other. (Study Session 4, LOS 13.l)

40. **B** A firm in a monopoly position will reduce output to where MC = MR, which will increase price, decrease consumer surplus, and increase producer surplus. A marginal cost pricing strategy refers to regulation which requires a firm to set price equal to marginal cost. (Study Session 4, LOS 16.d)

41. **A** Sales and purchases of non-financial assets in a country are accounted for in the capital account. (Study Session 6, LOS 20.g)

42. **A** The marginal cost curve intersects both the AVC and ATC curves at their minimum points. If the cost of producing the next unit of output (marginal cost) is less than the average cost (variable or total) of the units already produced, producing the next unit will decrease the average cost. If the marginal cost is greater than the average cost of units already produced, then producing another unit will increase the average cost. (Study Session 4, LOS 15.d)

43. **C** Money's function as a medium of exchange permits the indirect trade of goods and services, which greatly increases the efficiency of carrying out transactions compared to barter. Its function as a unit of account permits buyers and sellers to calculate how much a good or service is worth in terms of other goods and services. Money's function as a store of value allows the holder to save it, delaying consumption to a later time without reducing the amount he can consume. (Study Session 5, LOS 19.b)

44. **B** The fiscal policy multiplier is positive for government spending and negative for taxes. Increasing taxes will decrease aggregate demand. The balanced budget multiplier (for equal-sized increases in government spending and taxes) is positive but less than the multiplier for spending only. (Study Session 5, LOS 19.o)

45. **C** The supplementary schedules to the financial statements typically detail a company's various business segments. (Study Session 7, LOS 22.c)

46. **C** Assets = liabilities + contributed capital + beginning retained earnings + revenues – expenses – dividends. Assets = 350 + 175 + 125 + 400 – 300 – 10 = 740. Alternatively, assets = liabilities + equity, or $350 + $215 + $175 = $740. (Study Session 7, LOS 23.b)

47. **C** Investment property is defined under IFRS as property held for the purpose of earning rental income, capital appreciation, or both. Owner-occupied property is not classified as investment property. (Study Session 9, LOS 30.k)

48. **A** Taxable income is $145 million ($150 million pretax income – $25 million municipal interest + $35 million warranty expense – $15 million depreciation). Income tax payable = $58 million ($145 taxable income × 40%). (Study Session 9, LOS 31.d)

49. **B** If a firm reverses a writedown of inventory, IFRS requires the firm to disclose the circumstances of the reversal. Because IFRS reporting firms may not use the LIFO cost flow assumption, they do not need to disclose a LIFO reserve and will not experience the effects on income of an inventory liquidation (drawdown) that occur under LIFO. (Study Session 9, LOS 29.g and Study Session 10, LOS 33.d)

50. **B** IFRS and U.S. GAAP require retrospective restatement of financial statements for all periods shown in the company's financial report. (Study Session 8, LOS 25.e)

51. **B** In a finance lease, the principal portion of the lease payment is reported as an outflow from financing activities. The entire payment on an operating lease is CFO. (Study Session 9, LOS 32.h)

52. C Accrued expenses are expenses incurred but not yet paid or recorded at the statement date. Wage expense should have been accrued and the corresponding liability (wages payable) recognized. Without this accrual entry, net income and owners' equity are overstated, while liabilities are understated. (Study Session 7, LOS 23.d)

53. A The seller financing is a noncash transaction. Accordingly, Wichita's 20X8 cash flows are unaffected. The noncash transaction should be disclosed in the footnotes to the 20X8 cash flow statement. (Study Session 8, LOS 27.a)

54. A Subtracting goodwill from assets can help make the financial statements of a firm that has grown through acquisitions more comparable to those of a firm that has generated internal growth. To adjust cost of goods sold from a LIFO basis to a FIFO basis, an analyst should *subtract* the change in the LIFO reserve for the period. When calculating solvency ratios, an analyst should add the *present value* of a firm's disclosed operating lease obligations to the firm's liabilities and long-lived assets. (Study Session 10, LOS 35.e)

55. **B** The importance of reporting standards is that they ensure that financial reports are usable by a wide range of audiences, including analysts. Reporting standards limit the range of presentation formats and accounting methods but do not require all firms to use the same format or methods. Reporting standards do not eliminate management discretion in choosing methods and making estimates, so they do not fully prevent manipulation of financial results. (Study Session 7, LOS 24.a)

56. **B** Increasing residual values of plant and equipment would decrease depreciation expense and increase operating income. Decreasing the useful lives of plant and equipment would increase depreciation expense by depreciating these assets over a shorter period. Under IFRS, the firm cannot recognize revaluation above depreciated cost on the income statement. Increasing the book value of plant and equipment would also increase depreciation expense in subsequent periods. (Study Session 9, LOS 30.c,g and Study Session 10, LOS 33.b)

57. C When interest is capitalized, the expenditure is reported as an investing outflow. When expensed immediately, the expenditure is reported as an operating outflow. Thus, CFO is higher and CFI is lower when costs are capitalized. Capitalizing construction costs will result in higher fixed assets; thus, fixed asset turnover is lower (higher denominator). Construction interest is not reported as interest expense. Instead, interest, along with the other capitalized construction costs, is allocated to the income statement as depreciation expense. Thus, capitalizing costs will result in a higher interest coverage ratio (lower denominator). (Study Session 8, LOS 28.b, and Study Session 9, LOS 30.a)

58. C Large differences between the interest coverage and fixed charge coverage ratios suggest that Kovacs and Linwood have significant lease payments. The firms' debt-to-equity ratios most likely do not reflect these obligations. McDowell appears to rely less on leases. The most appropriate solvency ratio for comparing these firms is fixed charge coverage. Compared to the other two firms, McDowell is better able to cover its fixed charges with earnings. (Study Session 9, LOS 32.l)

59. **B** To compute cash collections from customers, begin with net sales from the income statement, subtract (add) any increase (decrease) in accounts receivable, and add (subtract) any increase (decrease) in unearned revenue. (Study Session 8, LOS 27.g)

60. **A** Current liabilities are obligations due within one year or the company's operating cycle, whichever is longer. With an operating cycle of two years, Magnus should classify as current any liabilities that must be settled in less than two years. (Study Session 8, LOS 26.d)

61. **B** Valuation allowances occur when the probability of utilizing deferred tax assets is in doubt. Deferred tax assets must be reduced by a valuation allowance to reflect the probability that they will never be used. (Study Session 9, LOS 31.g)

62. **B** Barnes' bond offering is issued at a discount (market rate > coupon rate). The amortization of the discount will be added to interest expense, thus making the reported expense greater than the $12 million coupon payment ($200 million × 6%). (Study Session 9, LOS 32.a,b)

63. **C** Both firms sold 110 units (100 units in beginning inventory + 60 units purchased – 50 units in ending inventory). Using FIFO, Harrelson's COGS is $1,080 [(100 units × $10) + (10 units × $8)]. Using LIFO Wilson's COGS is $1,080 [(10 units × $6) + (30 units × $12) + (20 units × $8) + (50 units × $10)]. (Study Session 9, LOS 29.c)

64. **C** Diluted EPS must be reported if a firm has any potentially dilutive securities outstanding. In this case, the security is antidilutive (£500,000 / 400,000 = £1.25, which is greater than basic EPS), and the firm will report that diluted EPS is equal to basic EPS. (Study Session 8, LOS 25.h)

65. **C** Determining a target value for a ratio is difficult, so a range of values may be more appropriate. Financial ratios are not useful when viewed in isolation and are only valid when compared to historical figures or peers. Comparing ratios between firms can be complicated by variations in accounting treatments used at each firm. (Study Session 8, LOS 28.a)

66. **B** Other comprehensive income includes unrealized gains and losses on available-for-sale securities, foreign currency translation gains and losses, minimum pension liability adjustments, and unrealized gains and losses on derivatives used for cash flow hedging.

    Unrealized gains and losses on available-for-trading securities are included in net income on the income statement. Losses due to expropriation of assets would be included in net income, either as an extraordinary item (U.S. GAAP only) or an unusual or infrequent item (IFRS or U.S. GAAP). (Study Session 8, LOS 25.l)

67. **B** The difference between the sale proceeds and the carrying value for a long-lived asset is reported on a firm's income statement as a gain or loss. The carrying value is the original value less accumulated depreciation. (Study Session 9, LOS 30.i)

68. **C** IFRS allows interest paid to be reported in either the operating or financing section of the cash flow statement. U.S. GAAP requires interest paid to be reported in the operating section of the cash flow statement. (Study Session 8, LOS 27.c)

69. **B** Preferred stock pays constant dividends into perpetuity. The price of preferred stock equals the present value of the preferred stock dividends:

$$\$20 = \frac{\$2}{k_{ps}}$$

Therefore, the cost of preferred stock capital equals:

$$k_{ps} = \frac{\$2}{\$20} = 0.10 = 10\%.$$

(Study Session 11, LOS 37.g)

70. **C** Mason should use a higher marginal cost of capital than Mammoth Industries to adjust for the semiconductor division's higher cash flow risk. (Study Session 11, LOS 37.e)

71. **A** The R&D expenditure is a sunk cost that should not be considered in the project's cash flows. The opportunity cost of the empty building in its next-best use should be considered in the project analysis. (Study Session 11, LOS 36.b)

72. **C** When a capital budget is limited, the available funds should be allocated among projects that are expected to increase the value of the firm by the greatest amount. The increase in firm value can be measured by the project's NPV. The firm should calculate the NPV of each project and find the mix that maximizes the increase in firm value and does not exceed the funds available for investment. (Study Session 11, LOS 36.c)

73. **B** An NPV profile is a plot of the relationship between the NPV (expected value added) of a project and the cost of capital used to discount future cash flows. (Study Session 11, LOS 36.e)

74. **C** The cash conversion cycle measures the amount of time it takes for the firm to turn the firm's cash investments in inventory back into cash. A high cash conversion cycle implies that the company has too much invested in working capital. (Study Session 11, LOS 40.b)

75. **B** The break point at which new debt will increase the marginal cost of capital is calculated as \$3 million (the level of debt when the cost will change) divided by the percent of debt in the capital structure (30%). Break point = \$3 million / 0.3 = \$10 million in total new capital. (Study Session 11, LOS 37.k)

76. **C** Significant experience in financial operations and accounting are beneficial qualities of a board member. Having current or previous executives of the firm on the board is likely to align the board with management and limit the board's independence. While prior experience on a board is important, having served for significant periods may mean that the board member is too closely allied with management. (Study Session 11, LOS 41.d)

77. **C** The company's inventory management has been getting worse while that of the industry is getting better. The industry inventory turnover rates can be calculated by dividing 365 by the number of days of inventory for each of the years given. Year 1: 365 / 50 = 7.3x. Year 2: 365 / 49 = 7.4x. Year 3: 365 / 48 = 7.6x. The company's number of days of inventory can be calculated by dividing 365 by the inventory turnover rate for each of the years given. Year 1: 365 / 8.3 = 44. Year 2: 365 / 8.1 = 45.1. Year 3: 365 / 7.6 = 48. (Study Session 11, LOS 40.f)

78. **B** The capital structure ratios are:

Debt to total capital = \$10 / \$40 = 25%
Equity to total capital = \$30 / \$40 = 75%

The formula for the WACC (if no preferred stock) is:

$WACC = w_d k_d(1 - t) + w_e kc_e$

where w_d is the percentage of operations financed by debt, we is the percentage of operations financed by equity, *t* is the marginal tax rate, k_d is the before-tax cost of debt, and k_{ce} is the cost of common equity.

WACC = 0.25(0.08)(0.60) + 0.75(0.12) = 0.102 = 10.2%.

(Study Session 11, LOS 37.a,b)

79. **C** Closed-end mutual fund shares can be purchased for market-determined prices. Hedge funds (which include market neutral funds) and wrap fee (separately managed) accounts typically require substantial minimum investment amounts. (Study Session 12, LOS 42.d)

80. **A** All portfolios on the CML include the same tangency portfolio of risky assets, except the intercept (all invested in risk-free asset). The tangency portfolio contains none of the risk-free asset and "borrowing portfolios" can be constructed with a negative allocation to the risk-free asset. Portfolios on the CML are efficient (well-diversified) and have no unsystematic risk. (Study Session 12, LOS 44.b,c)

81. **C** With a core-satellite approach, a majority of the assets are invested passively (in the "core" portfolio) with a smaller proportion in actively managed "satellite" portfolios. This reduces the likelihood of excessive trading and offsetting active positions. (Study Session 12, LOS 45.g)

82. **B** The equation for the capital asset pricing model is:

$E(R_i) = R_F + \beta_i[E(R_m) - R_F]$

Beta measures the sensitivity of the stock's returns to changes in the returns on the market portfolio and is a standardized measure of the stock's systematic or non-diversifiable risk. As indicated by the CAPM equation, the expected return for any stock is related to its beta. In contrast, unsystematic risk does not affect the CAPM expected return. Therefore, according to the CAPM, expected returns are identical for assets with identical betas. Stock X has identical systematic risk but greater unsystematic risk than Stock Y, resulting in greater total risk (standard deviation). (Study Session 12, LOS 44.f)

83. **A** The Markowitz framework assumes that all investors view risk as the variability of returns. The variability of returns is measured as the variance (or equivalently standard deviation) of returns. The capital asset pricing model (CAPM) employs beta as the measure of an investment's systematic risk. (Study Session 12, LOS 43.g)

84. **C** Covariance indicates the direction of the linear relationship (i.e., positive or negative) between two variables, but its magnitude does not directly indicate the strength of that relationship. If 0.91 was the correlation, rather than the covariance, it would indicate the monthly returns on these two stocks have a strong linear relationship. (Study Session 12, LOS 43.b)

85. **A** Style indexes measure the returns to strategies that are differentiated by market capitalization or by value versus growth. A sector index measures the returns for an industry sector such as financials. Although market capitalization is one of the criteria for inclusion in the index, this does not suggest the index is value weighted. (Study Session 13, LOS 47.h)

86. **B** A short seller owes the lender any dividends declared on the shorted stock. The short seller does not receive any dividends to reinvest. (Study Session 13, LOS 46.e)

87. **A** Both statements accurately describe the characteristics of a well-functioning securities market. Statement 1 describes informational efficiency. Statement 2 describes operational efficiency. (Study Session 13, LOS 46.k)

88. **B** In an informationally efficient market, prices are unbiased estimates of securities' intrinsic values. Therefore, active management cannot consistently generate positive risk-adjusted returns compared to a passive index strategy. Because transactions costs reduce its net return, an active strategy underperforms a passive index strategy on average over time. (Study Session 13, LOS 48.a)

89. **A** An increase in ROE results when earnings grow more (or fall less) in percentage terms than equity over a period. Consider a firm whose equity falls by 40% and earnings fall by 30% over a period. ROE increases from the prior period but book value and market value may both fall as a result. Investors' required rate of return on a firm's shares depends on the risk of the shares, which is not a function of ROE by itself. (Study Session 14, LOS 49.g)

90. **A** The expected (P_0 / E_1) ratio is: $\frac{P_0}{E_1} = \frac{D_1 / E_1}{k - g}$. Holding other factors constant, increasing (k – g) or decreasing (D_1 / E_1) leads to a decrease in P_0/E_1. Increasing g while holding k constant leads to an increase in P_0 / E_1. (Study Session 14, LOS 51.h)

91. **A** $D_1 = 0.5 \times (1.15) = 0.575$
$D_2 = 0.575 \times (1.15) = 0.661$
$D_3 = 0.661 \times (1.15) = 0.760$

$$P_3 = \frac{0.76 \times 1.08}{0.1 - 0.08} = \frac{0.821}{0.02} = 41.05$$

$$V = \frac{0.575}{1.10} + \frac{0.661}{(1.10)^2} + \frac{0.760 + 41.05}{(1.10)^3} = 32.48$$

$32.48 < $35.00, so George should not buy the stock. (Study Session 14, LOS 51.a,e)

92. **B** When computing any price-weighted index, the denominator must be adjusted to take stock splits into account. (Study Session 13, LOS 47.d)

93. **B** The new acquisition has likely changed the nature of Acquire's business so that historical information is not as relevant to the investment decision-making process. The most appropriate earnings multiple for analyzing Acquire is the forward price-to-earnings ratio. (Study Session 14, LOS 51.g)

94. **B** "Behind the market" refers to a buy order with a limit price less than the best bid, or a sell order with a limit price higher than the best ask. A limit order that is behind the market (i.e., an order to buy for less than the market price or sell for more than the market price) will not be filled unless the market price moves to the order's limit price. "Inside the market" refers to orders with limit prices between the best bid and best ask. "Aggressively priced" refers to a buy order with limit prices higher than the best ask or a sell order with a limit price lower than the best bid. Aggressively priced limit orders are most likely to be filled immediately. (Study Session 13, LOS 46.h)

95. **B** In general, firms in highly concentrated industries, industries with high barriers to entry, and industries experiencing undercapacity are more likely to have strong pricing power than firms in fragmented industries, industries with low barriers to entry, and industries experiencing overcapacity. (Study Session 14, LOS 50.g)

96. **C** Liquidity is generally supplied by dealers in a quote-driven market, by other traders in an order-driven market, and by brokers (who arrange the trades) and traders in a brokered market. (Study Session 13, LOS 46.j)

97. **C** Deferred-coupon bonds carry coupons, but the initial coupon payments are deferred for some period. The coupon payments accrue, at a compound rate, over the deferral period and are paid as a lump sum at the end of that period. After the initial deferment period has passed, these bonds pay regular coupon interest for the rest of the life of the issue (i.e., until the maturity date). Zero coupon bonds do not pay periodic interest. A step-up note has a coupon rate that increases on one or more specified dates during the note's life. (Study Session 15, LOS 52.b)

98. **C** Yield volatility affects the value of options embedded in a bond. The value of an option-free bond, such as a U.S. Treasury bond, is not affected by changes in expected interest rate volatility. (Study Session 15, LOS 53.n)

99. **B** The lowest duration bond will have the least exposure to rising yields. Bond B provides the most protection from the expected increase in interest rates. (Study Session 16, LOS 58.b,c)

100. **C** Credit enhancement mechanisms and special purpose vehicles relate to asset-backed securities. (Study Session 15, LOS 54.i)

101. **A** If the OAS is greater than the *Z*-spread, the option cost is negative, which means that a put option is embedded in the bond, allowing investors to put the bond back to the issuer. A callable bond will have a positive option cost and a *Z*-spread is greater than the OAS. The bond is acceptable for the portfolio since it has no call option. (Study Session 16, LOS 57.f)

102. **C** With zero inflation and no expected change, the expectations hypothesis would predict a flat yield curve. The liquidity preference theory would predict an upward sloping yield curve to reflect the increased risk of the longer time horizon. (Study Session 15, LOS 55.c)

103. **B** The bond with the least percentage price change will be the bond with the lowest interest rate risk. Higher coupons or shorter maturities decrease interest rate risk. The bond with only five years to maturity will have the lowest interest rate risk. The government bond would have less credit risk, but similar interest rate risk, compared to the 10-year corporate bond. (Study Session 15, LOS 53.c)

104. **A** If a Treasury security is undervalued based on prevailing Treasury spot rates, its cash flows are priced higher individually (as Treasury STRIPS) than the bond itself. The dealer can earn an arbitrage profit by buying the bond and selling the STRIPS. The information given does not indicate whether the bond is undervalued relative to other Treasury securities. (Study Session 16, LOS 56.f)

105. **C** The classifications "investment grade" and "non-investment grade" are based on ratings from recognized credit rating agencies. Bonds rated Baa3/BBB+ or higher are classified as investment grade, while bonds rated Ba1/BB+ or lower are classified as non-investment grade. However, an analyst should not rely exclusively on credit ratings to draw conclusions about the credit risk or loss severity of bond investments. (Study Session 16, LOS 59.d)

106. **B** The 3-year spot rate is the discount rate for a 3-year zero-coupon security. To eliminate any opportunity for arbitrage, the 3-year spot rate should equal the compounded equivalent of borrowing at expected forward rates:

3-year spot rate = $[(1 + 0.03)(1 + 0.065)^2]^{1/3} - 1 = 0.0532 = 5.32\%$.

Note that the answer can be approximated simply by averaging the 1-year rate and the 2-year forward rate one year from now: (3 + 6.5 + 6.5) / 3 = 5.33%. (Study Session 16, LOS 57.g)

107. **B** An embedded call option increases a bond's yield to maturity, so its nominal and zero-volatility spreads will be higher than its option-adjusted spread. The option cost is the difference between the OAS and the *Z*-spread, or 40 basis points. (Study Session 16, LOS 57.f)

108. **B** First, calculate the bond's effective duration as follows: (98.2 – 91.41) / (2 × 94.73 × 0.005) = 6.79 / 0.9473 = 7.17. The change in price would be: –7.17 × (–0.0075) × 94.73 = 5.09, for a new price of 94.73 + 5.09 = 99.82. (Study Session 16, LOS 58.d,e)

109. **C** If the bond was priced to yield 5.5%, it would trade at a premium and the current yield (annual coupon / bond price) would be less than 7%. Because Scott's reinvestment rate is below the yield to maturity of 6.25%, her actual return would be below 6.25%. Because the bond is currently priced at a premium (YTM < coupon), the yield to call is less than the yield to maturity, and the yield to worst would be less than 6.25% even if coupons were reinvested at 6.25%. (Study Session 16, LOS 57.b)

110. **C** Zero-coupon bonds (such as a Treasury STRIP) have no reinvestment risk over their lives but have a high degree of interest rate risk. The mortgage-backed security would have higher reinvestment risk due to the need to reinvest not only the coupon payments, but amortized principal payments as well. (Study Session 15, LOS 53.i)

111. **B** Neither statement is accurate. The maximum profit to a long call position is infinite since the value of the underlying stock can increase indefinitely. The maximum profit on a short call position is limited to the premium for which the option is sold. Since an infinite sum is always greater than a finite call premium, the maximum profit on a long call is always greater than the maximum profit on a short call. A long put position has a breakeven point equal to the strike price less the premium paid for the option. If the put option is at the money, the underlying stock price is equal to the strike price. The stock price must decrease by the amount of the premium before the breakeven point is reached. Ulrich stated that the stock must decrease by any amount to break even, which is incorrect. (Study Session 17, LOS 65.a)

112. **B** The intrinsic value of a put is the difference between strike price and stock price if stock price is less than strike price (80 – 78 = 2). The loss is equal to the intrinsic value minus the premium paid (2 – 5 = –3). (Study Session 17, LOS 63.h)

113. **A** Being long a call has limited downside risk, but an unlimited upside, just as a protective put position does. Covered calls have very limited upside potential and a long call-short put position has significant downside risk. (Study Session 17, LOS 65.b)

114. **B** The writer of an option on futures gives the option holder the right to take a short position in a futures contract. If the holder exercises the option, the option writer must take the long position in the futures contract. (Study Session 17, LOS 63.e)

115. **C** $S_0 = c_0 - p_0 + X / (1 + r)^T$

where:
c_0 = buy call current value
p_0 = buy put current value
S_0 = current stock price
X = exercise price
r = risk-free rate
T = time horizon

$S_0 = 4 - 2.25 + [50 / (1 + 0.02)]$

$S_0 = 50.77$

(Study Session 17, LOS 63.m)

116. **B** Burke's exposure to cotton is long since she already owns the asset and will need to sell it in the market at a future date. Therefore, she needs a short forward position to offset her price risk. Thus, Anderson has taken the long position in the forward contract. Since the contract is nondeliverable, it will be settled in cash upon the expiration date. At the time of expiration, the market price of cotton is $49 and the contract price is $47. This is a $2 gain to Anderson, the long position, who has the obligation to purchase the cotton for $47 but can immediately sell it for $49 in the market. Therefore, Burke owes Anderson $2. It is possible, however, that Burke will not have the funds or may simply refuse to fulfill her side of the contract. Therefore, Anderson has credit risk since there is no guarantee that Burke will pay. (Study Session 17, LOS 61.a)

117. **A** Hedge funds that employ a market neutral strategy maintain approximately equal values in long and short equity positions so that stock selection, rather than market exposure, determines their investment performance. (Study Session 18, LOS 66.d)

118. **A** Downside risk measures may be more appropriate than standard deviation for estimating risk of hedge funds, which often have leptokurtic and negatively skewed returns distributions. Standard deviation is typically an appropriate risk measure for publicly traded securities such as REITs and ETFs. (Study Session 18, LOS 66.g)

119. **B** Management fee = $100 million × 2.0% = $2.0 million

Incentive fee = [$110 million – $100 million – $2 million – ($100 million × 5.0%)] × 20% = $0.6 million

Total fee = $2.0 million + $0.6 million = $2.6 million

End-of-year value after fees = $110.0 – $2.60 = $107.4 million

Net return = ($107.4 million / $100.0 million) – 1 = 7.4%.

(Study Session 18, LOS 66.f)

120. **B** Positive roll yields occur when the market for a commodity is in backwardation. In a backwardated market, the futures price is less than the current spot price. Assuming the spot price remains unchanged, the futures price will increase over the life of the contract, and at expiration the futures price will equal the spot price.
(Study Session 18, LOS 67.a,b)

Exam 2
Morning Session Answers

To get valuable feedback on how your score compares to those of other Level I candidates, use your Username and Password to gain Online Access at schweser.com and choose the left-hand menu item "Practice Exams Vol. 2."

1. A	31. C	61. A	91. A
2. C	32. C	62. B	92. A
3. A	33. A	63. A	93. C
4. B	34. C	64. C	94. A
5. C	35. C	65. B	95. B
6. A	36. B	66. A	96. A
7. C	37. B	67. B	97. B
8. C	38. B	68. A	98. A
9. C	39. A	69. A	99. C
10. C	40. A	70. B	100. C
11. B	41. B	71. C	101. B
12. A	42. B	72. B	102. B
13. C	43. A	73. C	103. A
14. B	44. C	74. B	104. B
15. B	45. C	75. A	105. A
16. C	46. B	76. A	106. B
17. C	47. A	77. A	107. A
18. B	48. B	78. B	108. C
19. A	49. C	79. B	109. C
20. A	50. C	80. A	110. B
21. B	51. A	81. B	111. A
22. B	52. B	82. B	112. B
23. B	53. B	83. C	113. A
24. B	54. C	84. A	114. C
25. A	55. B	85. A	115. C
26. C	56. A	86. C	116. A
27. A	57. C	87. C	117. C
28. B	58. C	88. A	118. A
29. B	59. C	89. B	119. A
30. B	60. C	90. B	120. A

Exam 2
Morning Session Answers

Answers referencing the Standards of Practice address Study Session 1, LOS 1.b, c and 2.a, b, c, except where noted.

1. **A** Standard V(A) Diligence and Reasonable Basis does not require a Member to dissociate from a group recommendation, as long as the opinion has a reasonable and adequate basis.

2. **C** The enforcement structure for the Code and Standards is centered around the Rules of Procedure, which are based on two primary principles: fair process and confidentiality of proceedings. "Global application" relates to the Code and Standards. (Study Session 1, LOS 1.a)

3. **A** Standard III(D) Performance Presentation does not prohibit showing past performance of funds managed at a previous firm as part of a performance track record if accompanied by appropriate disclosures. In this instance, Arc clearly detailed that the performance occurred while Martin was the manager of Alpha Emerging Markets Fund. A minimum 5-year performance history is a requirement for GIPS compliance, but use of GIPS is not required by Standard III(D).

4. **B** An effective firewall includes a system for review by authorized compliance personnel of communications between departments on either side of the wall. Prohibiting any buying and selling is not recommended because doing so can provide a signal to other market participants; the firm should continue to execute unsolicited buy and sell orders from customers. Distribution of restricted lists should be limited to the compliance personnel responsible for monitoring trading in the restricted securities.

5. **C** According to Standard VII(B) Reference to CFA Institute, the CFA Designation, and the CFA Program, the CFA mark must not be used as a noun. It is acceptable to state that Wilson completed the examinations in consecutive years if this is true, but it is not acceptable to claim that this implies superior ability.

6. **A** According to Standard I(B) Independence and Objectivity, members must not accept any gift that may compromise their independence and objectivity. Because Welch has had a long-standing relationship with Orham Brokers, the symphony tickets have relatively small value, and Orham provides superior execution at competitive commission rates, it is unlikely that the symphony tickets will influence Welch's independence and objectivity. The gift does not raise a conflict of interest with Welch's employer that would require disclosure under Standard IV(B) Additional Compensation Arrangements. Therefore it is acceptable for Welch to accept the tickets without disclosure.

7. **C** Russ can make use of her opinions, so long as she distinguishes them from fact. The expected settlement is public information because the source is a newspaper quote. Russ may use this information but should cite the newspaper article.

8. **C** Liu violated Standard I(C) Misrepresentation because she included quotations from "investment experts" without specific reference to their source. Yang, however, did not violate the Standard because it permits members to use, without acknowledgment, factual information published by recognized financial and statistical reporting services, such as Standard & Poor's.

9. **C** According to Standard VI(A) Disclosure of Conflicts, members must prominently and clearly disclose to clients, prospects, and their employer, anything that could affect their independence and objectivity or interfere with their duties to those parties. As a beneficial owner of shares in Swift & Company, Roberts has incentive to increase the value of Swift stock for her personal gain, even though she is unaware of the actual amount or value of the trust holdings. This is a potential conflict of interest that must be disclosed to clients and employer.

10. **C** When a client submits an order to trade in a security on which the firm has changed its recommendation, Standard III(B) Fair Dealing requires members and candidates to advise the client of the recommendation change before accepting the order. Smith should not assume White received and read the e-mail that included the change in recommendation. Notifying clients is not the analyst's responsibility.

11. **B** Under Standard VI(A) Disclosure of Conflicts, members must make full and fair disclosure of all matters that could reasonably be expected to interfere with their independence or objectivity when dealing with clients. Disclosure of Anthony's new position in Abco will allow his clients the opportunity to judge Anthony's motives and potential biases for themselves.

12. **A** Management discussions with analysts are not considered public disclosure. It is likely that this information will have an impact on DM's stock price, thus it is considered to be material nonpublic information. Kelley and Gordon may not act or cause others to act on the information. They should encourage the firm's management to release this information to the public.

13. **C** Standard VI(C) Referral Fees requires members to disclose to their clients any compensation or benefit received for the recommendation of services. Full disclosure should be made in writing and should include the nature and value of the benefit. Disclosure of a compensation arrangement will allow the client to evaluate whether Lewis' recommendation of another department within Kite Brothers is influenced by the referral fee.

14. **B** Total firm assets include discretionary and non-discretionary assets, and include both fee-paying and non-fee paying accounts. When presenting GIPS-compliant composites, non-discretionary accounts are excluded. (Study Session 1, LOS 4.a)

15. **B** Brenner's actions comply with the conditions specified in Standard IV(B) Additional Compensation Arrangements. He notified his employer in writing (e-mail is acceptable) of the terms and conditions of additional compensation arrangement and received permission from his employer. Loyalties to other clients may be affected, but it is the employer's duty to determine this. Nothing in the Standard specifies that "all parties involved" includes other clients.

16. **C** Standard III(E) Preservation of Confidentiality suggests the most appropriate action is to check with compliance or legal counsel before going forward to the authorities regarding a possible violation. CFA Institute recognizes that in some cases there may be an obligation to not "preserve confidentiality" and disclose information as required by law. The activities described are only suspected, and proper care should be taken to not expose her firm to liability if confidential allegations of impropriety are improperly disclosed.

17. **C** After the employee has left the firm, his or her skills and knowledge while employed (including client names) are not considered confidential or privileged information.

18. **B** Standard VI(B) Priority of Transactions states that family accounts that are client accounts should be treated like other firm accounts and should not be given special treatment nor be disadvantaged due to a family relationship with the member.

19. **A** Look-ahead bias occurs when a study examines an effect based on information that was not yet available at the time being tested. In this case, year-end book values per share are not known until well into the first quarter of the following year.

    Time-period bias is present when a study covers either too short a period (the proposed relationship may only hold during that time frame) or too long a period (the proposed relationship may have changed during that span). Sample selection bias refers to taking a sample that is not representative of the population being studied. (Study Session 3, LOS 10.k)

20. **A** The paired comparisons test is performed using a *t*-statistic with n–1 degrees of freedom. (Study Session 3, LOS 11.h)

21. **B** Simply add the probabilities associated with the probability function for the categories 1,000, 1,500, and 2,000: 0.2 + 0.2+ 0.2 = 0.6. There is a 60% probability that unit demand will fall in the range of 1,000 to 2,000 units. (Study Session 2, LOS 7.c)

22. **B** To calculate the covariance, you first must calculate the expected returns (means) for each stock:

    Expected return for A-Marts: 0.35(0.20) + 0.50(0.04) + 0.15(–0.20) = 0.06

    Expected return for Shops R Us: 0.35(0.10) + 0.50(0.02) + 0.15(–0.10) = 0.03

    The covariance is the weighted average of the cross-products:

    Covariance = 0.35(0.20 – 0.06)(0.10 – 0.03) + 0.50(0.04 – 0.06)(0.02 – 0.03) + 0.15(–0.20 – 0.06)(–0.10 – 0.03)

    Covariance = 0.35(0.14)(0.07) + 0.50(–0.02)(–0.01) + 0.15(–0.26)(–0.13) = 0.0086 (Study Session 2, LOS 8.k)

23. **B** The money-weighted rate of return is the internal rate of return that makes the present value of cash outflows equal to the present value of cash inflows. From the investors' standpoint, the only cash outflow is the original \$10 million. The cash flows to the investors are \$500,000 + \$2,000,000 at year 1, and \$400,000 + \$9,000,000 at year 2.

Therefore, the money-weighted return is the value of r that solves:

$$10{,}000{,}000 = \frac{2{,}500{,}000}{(1+r)} + \frac{9{,}400{,}000}{(1+r)^2}$$

The money-weighted return (internal rate of return) can be found by using the following functions on the calculator:

$CF_0 = -10{,}000{,}000$
$CF_1 = 2{,}500{,}000$
$CF_2 = 9{,}400{,}000$

Then compute IRR, which equals 10.256%. (Study Session 2, LOS 6.d)

24. **B** Chebyshev's inequality states that, for any set of observations, regardless of the distribution of the data (skewed or not), the percentage of observations that lie within *k* standard deviations of the mean is at least $1 - (1/k^2)$. The central limit theorem applies as sample sizes get large and is inappropriate for a sample size of 20 or less from a non-normal distribution. (Study Session 2, LOS 7.h)

25. **A** A zero percent return lies 2 standard deviations below the mean return. Because these returns are normally distributed, 95% of the returns lie within 2 standard deviations of the mean, or from 0% to 20%. There is a 5% probability that the return will be either below 0% or above 20%, and by the symmetry property, there is a 2.5% probability that the return will lie below 0%. (Study Session 3, LOS 9.l)

26. **C** The strongest statement we can make is that the sample does not provide evidence that would lead us to reject the null hypothesis at the chosen significance level. We do not accept the null hypothesis, we only fail to reject it. We cannot conclude from the information given whether most sampled returns are greater than the market return. (Study Session 3, LOS 11.a)

27. **A** The unconditional probability that the economy will enter a recession is determined using the total probability rule, which is expressed by the following equation:

P(R) = P(recession and interest rates increase) or P(recession and no interest rate increase)

$P(R) = P(R \text{ and } I) + P(R \text{ and } I^c)$

$P(R) = P(R|I)P(I) + P(R|I^c)P(I^c)$

(Study Session 2, LOS 8.e)

28. **B** The efficient markets hypothesis, which holds that all available information is reflected in current security prices, is the major challenge to technical analysis. (Study Session 3, LOS 12.a)

29. **B** The cumulative distribution function gives the probability that a random variable will be less than or equal to a certain value. At \$35, the cumulative distribution function is 88%, which indicates that there is an 88% probability that the stock price will be less than or equal to \$35. (Study Session 3, LOS 9.d)

30. **B** PV = 500,000; N = 12; PMT = 12,700 ; FV = –2,000,000; CPT → I/Y = 11%. (Study Session 2, LOS 5.e,f)

31. **C** The distribution is positively skewed, therefore mean > median > mode. (Study Session 2, LOS 7.j,k)

32. **C** The effective annual yield (EAY) will always be greater than the bond-equivalent yield (BEY) because the EAY compounds the semiannual interest rate, while the bond equivalent yield does not. The relationship between EAY and BEY can be demonstrated by algebra:

    BEY = 2 × Semiannual Yield

    EAY = (1 + Semiannual Yield)^2 – 1 = 2 × Semiannual Yield + Semiannual Yield^2

    EAY = BEY + Semiannual Yield^2

    (Study Session 2, LOS 6.f)

33. **A** Because a profit-maximizing firm produces the quantity for which marginal cost equals marginal revenue, marginal cost must equal 25. Average revenue (i.e., price) of 12,000 / 300 = 40 is greater than marginal revenue, therefore the firm earns an economic profit. Because marginal cost is less than price the firm must face a downward sloping demand curve. We cannot conclude that an increase in productive capacity will increase profits. (Study Session 4, LOS 15.a,b)

34. **C** Because the real money supply is held constant in constructing each LM curve, holding the nominal money supply constant and changing the price level results in a new LM curve with a different real money supply. The intersections of the IS curve with LM curves at each price level illustrate a negative relationship between the price level and real income, i.e., the aggregate demand curve. (Study Session 5, LOS 17.f)

35. **C** Placing a tariff on an imported good increases the good's domestic price, which reduces the quantity demanded. However, the quantity supplied by domestic firms increases with the domestic equilibrium price, as does producer surplus for domestic firms. (Study Session 6, LOS 20.e)

36. **B** If the GDP deflator is 106.5, the price level has increased 6.5% since the base period and nominal GDP is 6.5% greater than real GDP. Because the base period is not necessarily the previous year, we cannot conclude that 6.5% is the annual inflation rate. (Study Session 5, LOS 17.c)

37. **B** Greater pricing power for the individual firm and a high concentration ratio suggest Product S is produced in an oligopolistic industry. Product T, with less pricing power for firms and a lower concentration ratio, is most likely producted by an industry characterized by monopolistic competition. (Study Session 4, LOS 16.g,h)

38. **B** Under the elasticities approach, currency depreciation will result in greater improvement in the trade deficit when either import or export demand becomes more elastic. One shortcoming of the elasticities approach is that it considers trade flows and ignores capital flows. The absorption approach considers both. Under the absorption approach, depreciation of the domestic currency will improve the balance of trade if it increases domestic savings (i.e., increases national income relative to expenditures). (Study Session 6, LOS 21.i)

39. **A** All firms maximize profits at the point where marginal revenue equal marginal cost. For a monopolist, this occurs at a lower output level than for a purely competitive firm, because the monopolist has a marginal revenue curve that falls below the demand curve, while the purely competitive firm has a marginal revenue curve that lies along the demand curve. (Study Session 4, LOS 16.a,b,d)

40. **A** The real exchange rate increased from 2.50 PTR/BAL to (3.00 PTR/BAL × 110/120) = 2.75 PTR/BAL. Note that the real exchange rate at the base period is equal to the nominal exchange rate because the CPIs are both 100 for the base period. The purchasing power of one PTR worth of domestic goods has decreased. When the real exchange rate (expressed as d/f) increases, exports of goods and services become relatively less expensive. (Study Session 6, LOS 21.a)

41. **B** An increase in the quantity of money at full employment will reduce interest rates in the short run, which would increase short-run aggregate demand above full employment. This causes wage demands to increase, which in turn reduces short-run aggregate supply. In the long run, real GDP reverts to its full-employment level with an increase in price level equal to the percentage increase in the quantity of money. (Study Session 5, LOS 17.i, 19.j)

42. **B** If the demand curve is less elastic than the supply curve, consumers will bear a higher portion of the tax burden. Suppliers will bear a greater portion of the tax burden if demand is more elastic than supply. Consumers and suppliers will share in the tax burden equally if the elasticity of supply equals the elasticity of demand. (Study Session 4, LOS 13.j,k)

43. **A** Selling government securities on the open market reduces bank reserves and drives up the federal funds rate. The other two statements are incorrect because the Federal Reserve does not directly control exchange rates or the prices of government securities. (Study Session 5, LOS 19.h)

44. **C** Unemployment due to workers lacking the necessary skills for a changing job market is called structural unemployment. Gold will likely seek work elsewhere as a bookkeeper. There was no broad economic downturn that would suggest cyclical unemployment. This is an example of frictional unemployment. (Study Session 5, LOS 18.d)

45. **C** Management prepares the financial statements, not the auditor. Verification of inventory amounts is not a main objective. Auditors selectively verify some items. (Study Session 7, LOS 22.d)

46. **B** The distribution of dividends to shareholders is considered a financing cash flow under U.S. GAAP. (Study Session 8, LOS 27.c)

47. **A** With increasing prices, the FIFO method would have reported a higher inventory balance compared to the LIFO method. The higher inventory level would produce a higher working capital balance. (Study Session 8, LOS 25.d)

48. **B** Double declining balance:

$$\text{Depreciation in Year i} = \frac{2}{n} \times (\text{Original cost} - \text{accumulated depreciation})$$

$$\text{Year 1} = \frac{2}{10}(550{,}000 - 0) = 110{,}000$$

$$\text{Year 2} = \frac{2}{10}(550{,}000 - 110{,}000) = 88{,}000$$

(Study Session 8, LOS 25.d)

49. **C** $\left[100{,}000 \times 2 \times \left(\frac{5}{12}\right)\right] + \left[80{,}000 \times 2 \times \left(\frac{7}{12}\right)\right] = 176{,}666$. There are 100,000 shares outstanding for the first five months of the year and 80,000 shares outstanding for seven months of the year, which must both be multiplied by 2 to reflect the stock split and by the fraction of the year for which the number of shares outstanding is applicable. (Study Session 8, LOS 25.g)

50. **C** Unrealized gains and losses on securities classified as available-for-sale are recorded as increases (gains) or decreases (losses) in other comprehensive income. Unrealized gains and losses on actively traded securities would be reported in the income statement. (Study Session 8, LOS 25.l)

51. **A** Under U.S. GAAP, research and development costs are not permitted to be recorded as intangible assets. They must be expensed against income as they occur. (Study Session 8, LOS 26.e)

52. **B** The IASB is a standard-setting body that is responsible for establishing financial reporting standards. The SEC is a regulatory authority, and IOSCO is an organization of regulatory authorities. (Study Session 7, LOS 24.b)

53. **B** A purchased, identifiable intangible asset with a finite life is amortized over its useful life. Costs incurred to develop an intangible asset such as a trademark are expensed when incurred. A patent that expires in the current period will not provide future benefits and therefore should not be recognized as an asset. (Study Session 9, LOS 30.b)

54. **C** An analyst can use the information in the details of debt repayment schedules in the footnotes and management's commentary to determine the timing and amount of future cash outflows necessary for the firm to make scheduled principal payments on its debt. The market value of outstanding debt is not typically included in the disclosures. Balance sheet values of debt and/or market value of debt, together with information about assets, provide information about leverage. (Study Session 9, LOS 32.e)

55. **B** The repayment of long-term debt is reported as a financing activity on the cash flow statement. Conversion of debt to equity and this particular asset acquisition are noncash transactions, which must be disclosed in the footnotes. (Study Session 8, LOS 27.b)

56. **A** The change in assets must be balanced by an equal change in liabilities and equity. If cash decreases by $10,000, and inventories increase by $13,000, the net change in assets is an increase of $3,000. An increase of $3,000 in accounts payable, a liability, keeps the accounting equation in balance. Neither of the other choices results in a balanced accounting equation. (Study Session 7, LOS 23.c)

57. **C** A company negotiating a new labor contract is likely to understate earnings to get a more favorable contract. By expensing rather than capitalizing costs, the company will reduce its reported net income. LIFO liquidation at year-end will result in a lower COGS and higher net income, offset by higher tax expense. By deferring expenses, the company will report higher net income. (Study Session 10, LOS 33.a)

58. **C** The difference between FCFF and FCFE equals the sum of net borrowing during the period and interest expense net of tax.

    FCFF = CFO + interest expense × (1 – tax rate) – fixed capital investment

    FCFE = CFO – fixed capital investment + net borrowing

    FCFF – FCFE = interest expense × (1 – tax rate) – net borrowing

    (Study Session 8, LOS 27.i)

59. **C** Since the fair value of Raider ($400,000) exceeds the carrying value of Raider ($385,000 including goodwill), no impairment exists; thus, no gain or loss is recognized. (Study Session 9, LOS 30.h)

60. **C** The interest income from municipal bonds is a permanent difference; thus, no deferred taxes are created and the difference is reflected in the company's effective tax rate. The different depreciation methods result in temporary differences that are expected to reverse. In the case of depreciation, a deferred tax liability is created. Valuation allowance accounts only apply to deferred tax assets and are created when it becomes probable that the company will not have enough future income to realize the full value of the deferred tax assets. (Study Session 9, LOS 31.f)

61. **A** Assets provide probable future economic benefits, are controlled by an entity, and are the result of previous transactions. Liabilities represent obligations owed by an entity from previous transactions. Stockholders' equity is the residual interest in assets after subtracting liabilities. (Study Session 8, LOS 26.a)

62. **B** Issuing common stock would increase shareholders' equity. Dividends received are included in net income and retained earnings. Realized gains on available-for-sale securities are also included in net income, and if any unrealized gains on these securities had been recognized previously as other comprehensive income, they would be removed from accumulated other comprehensive income when the firm realized the gains. (Study Session 8, LOS 26.g)

63. **A** If two of the criteria in a stock screen are dependent in some way, a stock that passes the first criterion is more likely to pass the second, dependent criterion than it would be to pass a different, independent criterion. Thus, dependence among the criteria tends to increase the number of stocks that satisfy all the criteria and "pass through" the screen. (Study Session 10, LOS 35.d)

64. **C** Debt is unaffected by the use of operating leases, while debt increases with the use of finance leases. The debt to equity ratio is lower using operating leases. Interest expense is unaffected by the use of operating leases, while interest expense increases with the use of finance leases. Interest coverage is generally higher when operating leases are used. A company using operating leases generally has a higher return on assets because of the lower reported asset base. (Study Session 9, LOS 32.h,l)

65. **B** Under IFRS, if a company recognizes a loss because the net realizable value of inventory has decreased below its historical cost, the company may revalue the inventory upward and recognize a gain (up to the amount of the previous loss) if the value of the inventory recovers. U.S. GAAP does not permit inventory to be revalued upward. (Study Session 9, LOS 29.f)

66. **A** Because prices are decreasing, FIFO ending inventory will be lower than LIFO ending inventory. There are 600 units remaining in ending inventory (2,700 units available – 2,100 units sold). Under LIFO, ending inventory is $30,000 (600 units × $50) and under FIFO, ending inventory is $27,600 (600 units × $46 per unit). Thus, FIFO will result in lower ending inventory of $2,400 ($30,000 LIFO inventory – $27,600 FIFO inventory). (Study Session 9, LOS 29.c,e)

67. **B** Return on common equity is equal to (Net income – Preferred dividends) / Average common equity.

20X8 preferred dividends = $12.5 million × 8% = $1 million.

20X7 common equity = $3 million common stock + 30 million additional paid-in-capital + $75 million retained earnings – $4 million treasury stock = $104 million.

20X8 common equity = $4 million common stock + $40 million additional paid-in-capital + $88 million retained earnings – $4 million treasury stock = $128 million.

Average common equity = ($104 million + $128 million) / 2 = $116 million.

Return on common equity = ($14 million 20X8 net income – $1 million preferred dividend) / $116 million average common equity = 11.2%.

(Study Session 8, LOS 28.b)

68. **A** ROE can be broken out as:

ROE = Tax burden × Interest burden × EBIT Margin × Asset Turnover × Leverage
Prior Year: 0.15 = 0.60 × 0.80 × 0.26 × 1.06 × Leverage
Current Year: 0.14 = 0.62 × 0.81 × 0.26 × 1.06 × Leverage

Solving the equation for leverage reveals that the measure has decreased from 1.13 in the prior year to 1.01 in the current year. This indicates Bivac is using less debt in its capital structure and is the most likely reason the company's ROE has declined.

The company's net profit margin has increased:

Net profit margin (Prior Year): 0.60 × 0.80 × 0.26 = 0.12
Net profit margin (Current Year): 0.62 × 0.81 × 0.26 = 0.13

The company's tax rate has decreased from 0.40 = (1 – 0.60) to 0.38 = (1 – 0.62). (Study Session 8, LOS 28.d)

69. **A** Capital rationing, or prioritizing projects to maximize the increase in company value, is necessary when the firm only has a limited amount of funds to invest. Project sequencing involves more than one project sequenced over time, and an unfavorable outcome for one project can cause cancellation of the next project in the sequence. Capital preservation is an investment return objective that involves an investment return at least equal to the inflation rate with minimal chance of loss. (Study Session 11, LOS 36.c)

70. **B** Greenmail refers to repurchasing shares at a premium to their market value by direct negotiation with a potential acquirer of the firm. (Study Session 11, LOS 39.c, 41.g)

71. **C** The NPV method implicitly assumes that cash flows can be reinvested at the project's cost of capital, while the IRR method assumes reinvestment at the computed IRR. (Study Session 11, LOS 36.e)

72. **B** Good corporate governance seeks to ensure that the firm acts lawfully and ethically in dealings with shareholders. The board of directors should protect shareholder interests, not management interests. The board should act independently of management, not as one with management. (Study Session 11, LOS 41.a)

73. **C** Changes in the tax rate would not affect the cost of equity for either company. If two companies have the same capital structure (i.e., equal weights of debt and equity) and have the same pretax component costs of capital (i.e., equal costs of debt and equity) they will have the same weighted average cost of capital (WACC) only if the companies have the same marginal tax rate. If one company has a higher tax rate, the after-tax cost of debt, $k_d(1 - t)$, will be lower and the WACC, $w_e k_e + w_d k_d(1 - t)$, will be lower as well. Beta Corporation has a lower current WACC since it has a higher tax rate. If Alpha's tax rate increases, its after-tax cost of debt will decrease and its WACC will decrease. (Study Session 11, LOS 37.b)

74. **B** $P_p = \frac{D_p}{r_p} = \frac{2.5}{0.0625} = 40.00$ (Study Session 11, LOS 37.g)

75. **A** Requiring that investors attend an annual meeting in order to vote shares limits their ability to vote. Confidential voting is supported by having third parties tabulate votes and by having the tabulation subject to audit. Cumulative voting typically may be viewed as supportive of shareholders' interests. (Study Session 11, LOS 41.g)

76. **A** Net operating cycle is calculated as the number of days of inventory + number of days of receivables – number of days of payables. Company Y's net operating cycles were 33 + 14 – 18 = 29 days in year 1 and 24 + 12 – 20 = 16 days in year 2. The decline in net operating cycle days in year 2 indicates an improvement in liquidity. For Company X, the net operating cycle for year 2 was 22 + 16 – 20 = 18 days, an increase from year 1, which was 18 + 14 – 19 = 13 days. (Study Session 11, LOS 40.c)

77. **A** The portfolio yield is a weighted average of the yields of the investments that comprise the portfolio. The weights are calculated as the value of each investment relative to the total portfolio value. The bond equivalent yields of the bank investments are given. For the U.S. Treasury bill, the bond-equivalent yield is:

(face value – market value) / market value × 365 / 90
= ($1,000,000 – 990,390) / 990,390 × 365 / 90 = 0.0097 × 0.04056 = 3.93%.

The total market value of the portfolio is $990,390 + $100,000 + $200,000 = $1,290,390. The portfolio yield equals:

3.93% ($990,390 / $1,290,390) + 4.34% ($100,000 / $1,290,390) + 4.84% ($200,000 / $1,290,390) = 4.10%, which is greater than the yield on the benchmark portfolio. (Study Session 11, LOS 40.e)

78. **B** The larger the company size, the more likely a firm is to use NPV for capital budgeting decisions. Private companies as well as companies located in European countries tend to use the payback period method more often than NPV or IRR. (Study Session 11, LOS 36.f)

79. **B** In a situation where the client's expressed willingness to bear investment risk is significantly less than the client's ability to bear investment risk, it is appropriate for the advisor to educate the client about investment risk and attempt to correct any misconceptions. It is not appropriate to attempt to change the investor's attitudes about risk in general or to change the investor's personality traits that lead to a low willingness to bear risk. (Study Session 12, LOS 45.d)

80. **A** The theoretical market portfolio used to form the capital market line (CML) is a market weighted global portfolio of all risky assets in existence. Since this portfolio contains all assets, it is well diversified. (Study Session 12, LOS 44.b)

81. **B** A stock with an expected return less than its required return is overvalued and will plot below the security market line (SML). A stock with an expected return equal to its required return is fairly valued and will plot on the SML. A stock with an expected return greater than its required return is undervalued and will plot above the SML. (Study Session 12, LOS 44.h)

82. **B** Returns on major asset classes have exhibited negative skewness (which reflects larger and more frequent negative deviations from their mean returns than a normal distribution) and positive excess kurtosis (which reflects larger and more frequent positive and negative deviations from their mean returns than a normal distribution). (Study Session 12, LOS 43.c)

83. **C** The covariance equals the product of the correlation and the two standard deviations. The standard deviation for Lumber Providers is $\sqrt{0.16} = 0.40$ and for Smithson Homebuilders is $\sqrt{0.25} = 0.50$. Therefore, covariance $= -0.60 \times (0.40) \times (0.50) = -0.12$. (Study Session 12, LOS 43.e)

84. **A** As stocks are randomly added to a portfolio, unsystematic risk decreases. A well-diversified 20-stock portfolio has little unsystematic risk. (Study Session 12, LOS 44.c)

85. **A** An operationally efficient market is characterized by low trading costs. The low trading costs of an operationally efficient market will encourage trading based on new information, thus making security prices more informationally efficient. High trading costs limit traders' ability to exploit violations of informational efficiency. (Study Session 13, LOS 46.k)

86. **C** Other things equal, callable securities are riskier to the investor than non-callable securities, while putable securities are less risky than non-putable securities. Cumulative preference shares are less risky than non-cumulative preference shares because cumulative shares are entitled to receive any missed dividend payments before the firm may pay a common dividend. (Study Session 14, LOS 49.e)

87. **C** The dividend can be of any size. Suppose it is $1.00.

The purchase price is 1.00 / 0.06 = 16.667.

The sale price is 1.00 / 0.05 = 20.

Kim pays 16.667 and receives 20.00 plus a 1.00 dividend one year later. The rate of return is $[(20 + 1)/16.667] - 1 = 26\%$. (Study Session 14, LOS 51.d)

88. **A** Data mining bias results from the likelihood that some statistically significant relationships will show up by chance in a large enough number of tests. A test at the 5% significance level of the hypothesis that stock prices are not correlated with a variable will reject about 1 such hypothesis in 20 when the hypothesis is true. (Study Session 13, LOS 48.f)

89. **B** The Dow Jones Industrial Average is a price-weighted index. If each of its stocks changes by the same percentage, the stock with the largest impact on the index will be the one with the highest price per share. (Study Session 13, LOS 47.d,k)

90. **B** In a call market, stocks trade at specific times at one price that clears the market for the stock. In continuous markets, trades occur at any time the market is open at prices set by auction or by dealer quotes. (Study Session 13, LOS 46.j)

91. **A** g = ROE × retention rate = [16.68 / 115] × [1 – (7.5 / 16.68)] = 0.145 × (1 – 0.45) = 7.975%. This growth rate represents the rate at which a company can grow its equity using internally generated funds. (Study Session 14, LOS 51.e)

92. **A** In a weak-form efficient market, market prices incorporate all market related information. In a semistrong-form efficient market, market prices incorporate all market and non-market public information. In a strong-form efficient market, market prices incorporate all market, non-market public, and private information. Positive risk-adjusted returns for specialists indicate that this market is not strong-form efficient as specialists have access to non-public information. Slow price adjustment to earnings surprises suggest this market is not semistrong-form efficient. (Study Session 13, LOS 48.d)

93. **C** required return = RFR + β [R_m – RFR]

equity risk premium = [R_m – RFR]

required return = 0.03 + 1.5 [0.06] = 0.12. (Study Session 14, LOS 51.e)

94. **A** Industry rotation is an active management strategy of overweighting or underweighting industries, compared to their strategic allocation weights, based on the stage of the business cycle. (Study Session 14, LOS 50.a)

95. **B** Futures contracts are standardized contracts traded on an exchange that obligate one party to purchase and one party to sell a specific amount of an asset at a specified price on a specified future date. Forward contracts are similar to futures contracts but are customizable (i.e., not standardized) and traded over-the-counter (i.e., not exchange-traded). Call options can be traded on an exchange; however, they give the holder the right, not the obligation, to purchase the asset at a future date. (Study Session 13, LOS 46.c and Study Session 17, LOS 60.a,c)

96. **A** $\frac{P_0}{E_1} = \frac{D_1 / E_1}{k - g} = \frac{1 - 0.6}{0.1 - 0.05} = 8.$

(Study Session 14, LOS 51.h)

97. **B** A nonrefundable bond is one that may not be redeemed with the proceeds from a new issue with a lower coupon. The bond may be redeemed with funds from other sources. Refund protection does not imply call protection. (Study Session 15, LOS 52.d)

98. **A** First we compute the yield to maturity of the bond. PV = –\$958.97, FV = \$1,000, PMT = ((4.2% × 1000) / 2 =) 21, n = (6 × 2 =)12, solve for i. I = 2.5%, multiply by 2 since it is a semiannual bond to get an annualized yield to maturity of 5.0%. Now compute the price of the bond at using yield one basis point higher, or 5.01%. FV = \$1,000, PMT = 21, n = 12, i = (5.01 / 2 =) 2.505, solve for PV. PV = –\$958.47. The price changes from \$958.97 to \$958.47, or \$0.50. (Study Session 16, LOS 58.j)

99. **C** Perry accurately stated the three steps in valuing a bond. Klein is incorrect regarding estimating the cash flows. When estimating cash flows, both principal and interest payments should be considered. (Study Session 16, LOS 56.a)

100. **C** Because Bond X has a coupon rate that is below the required yield, it will trade at a discount to par. Bond Y, with a coupon rate greater than the required yield, will trade at a premium to par. The fact that both bonds were issued at premiums does not matter, nor does the difference in time to maturity. (Study Session 15, LOS 53.b)

101. **B** Structured notes are medium-term notes that are combined with derivatives (options, futures, swaps, etc.). (Study Session 15, LOS 54.h)

102. **B** Effective duration should be used to measure interest rate for securities with embedded options (CMOs have a prepayment option). Convexity measures by themselves are not good measures of interest rate risk. (Study Session 16, LOS 58.f)

103. **A** If expected volatility increases, the value of the call option embedded in a callable bond will increase, thus lowering the value of the bond. $P_{\text{callable bond}} = P_{\text{non callable bond}}$ – call option. Likewise, the value of a put option will increase, increasing the value of the putable bond. $P_{\text{putable bond}} = P_{\text{nonputable bond}}$ + put option. (Study Session 15, LOS 53.n)

104. **B** The liquidity preference theory states that investors require a risk premium to hold longer term bonds. According to the liquidity preference theory, if short-term future expected interest rates are constant, the Treasury yield curve will be upward sloped. (Study Session 15, LOS 55.c)

105. **A** A security with a higher coupon rate will have higher reinvestment risk than a comparable security with a lower coupon rate. Interest rate risk (duration) is higher for the lower-coupon security. (Study Session 15, LOS 54.b)

106. **B** $(1.04^5 / 1.032^2)^{1/3} - 1 = 4.5\%$ (Study Session 16, LOS 57.g)

107. **A** Using the 10% yield to maturity, the price of the bond originally is \$754.22:
N = 10; I/Y = 10; PMT = 60; FV=1000; CPT PV = \$754.22

Using the 14% yield to maturity, the price of the bond changes to \$582.71:
N = 10; I/Y = 14; PMT = 60; FV=1000; CPT PV = \$582.71

Therefore, the price is expected to change from \$754.22 to \$582.71, a decrease of \$171.51. (Study Session 16, LOS 56.e)

108. **C** The impact on return will be greatest for the bond with the highest duration. For a 25 basis point (0.0025) increase in spread, the convexity adjustment is unlikely to be large enough to affect the ordering.

Calculations for each answer choice are as follows:

Return impact = –4(0.0025) + (1/2)(24)(0.0025)^2 = –0.99%

Return impact = –5(0.0025) + (1/2)(32)(0.0025)^2 = –1.24%

Return impact = –6(0.0025) + (1/2)(90)(0.0025)^2 = –1.47%

(Study Session 16, LOS 59.i)

109. **C** As rates fall, the option becomes more valuable, and the price of Bond X will not appreciate as rapidly as the noncallable Bond Y. The negative convexity of the callable bond will limit its price appreciation potential. (Study Session 15, LOS 53.d)

110. **B** To compute the value of this bond, discount each of the cash flows at a different interest rate appropriate for the timing of the cash flow. The appropriate rates are 40 bp greater than the Treasury yields.

$$\frac{40}{(1+0.044)}+\frac{40}{(1+0.049)^2}+\frac{(40+1,000)}{(1+0.0515)^3}=969.22.$$

(Study Session 16, LOS 57.e,f)

111. **A** This call option is in the money (€34 > €30). The lower bound on an in-the-money call option is the same [S – X / (1 + RFR)^T] for both American style and European style calls. (Study Session 17, LOS 63.j)

112. **B** Acting as the counterparty for all buyers and sellers is the primary role of the clearinghouse. By providing liquidity, the clearinghouse may also help lower transaction costs indirectly. (Study Session 17, LOS 62.a)

113. **A** A 2 × 8 FRA means that in 60 days (2 months), Grass will need to borrow the $12 million, and the agreement is based on 180-day (6 month) LIBOR.

$$\text{Transaction gain(loss)} = (12{,}000{,}000)\left(\frac{(0.06-0.06)\left(\frac{180}{360}\right)}{1+(0.06)\left(\frac{180}{360}\right)}\right)=0$$

(Study Session 17, LOS 61.f,g)

114. **C** $P = C + \left[X \big/ (1 + RFR)^T\right] + PV_{CF} - S_0$

$$P = 3.50 + \left[70 \big/ (1+0.053)^{3/12}\right] + \left(\frac{0.56}{(1+0.053)^{3/12}}\right) - 64 = 9.15$$

(Study Session 17, LOS 63.m,n)

115. **C** Interest rates have a direct relationship with call options and an inverse relationship with put options. Using these relationships, we can deduce that the increase in put option prices could have occurred as a result of a decrease in interest rates. Volatility is directly related to the price of all options (put or call). As volatility increases, so does the potential upside and downside prices of the underlying. The increase in the price of Merchant call options could have occurred as a result of increased volatility in Merchant stock. (Study Session 17, LOS 63.o)

116. **A**

Fixed rate payment is $50M × 0.07 × (91 / 365) =	$872,603
Equity payment is $50M × (1755 / 1825 – 1) =	$1,917,808
Total payment	$2,790,411

The negative equity payment increases the amount due from SingleSol. (Study Session 17, LOS 64.b)

117. **C** Convenience yield is the value of a physical commodity being available for use over the period of a futures contract. (Study Session 18, LOS 66.e)

118. **A** Management fee = €150 million × 2% = €3.0 million.

Incentive fee = [€150 million – €125 million – €3.0 million – (0.10 × €125 million)] × 20% = €1.9 million.

Total fee is €3.0 million + €1.9 million = €4.9 million. (Study Session 18, LOS 66.f)

119. **A** The seed stage is the earliest stage of a business and may involve funding research and development. The next stage of a business is known as the early stage and consists of financing of initial production and sales. The angel investing stage precedes the seed stage and involves planning based on new ideas for businesses. (Study Session 18, LOS 66.d)

120. **A** Appraisal index returns are based on estimates of property values and therefore tend to be smoother than repeat sales index returns, which are based on actual sale prices of properties. As a result, appraisal index returns have lower standard deviations. (Study Session 18, LOS 66.e)

Exam 2
Afternoon Session Answers

To get valuable feedback on how your score compares to those of other Level I candidates, use your Username and Password to gain Online Access at schweser.com and choose the left-hand menu item "Practice Exams Vol. 2."

1. A
2. A
3. B
4. A
5. A
6. A
7. A
8. C
9. B
10. A
11. B
12. B
13. C
14. C
15. A
16. A
17. C
18. B
19. B
20. B
21. A
22. B
23. B
24. B
25. A
26. A
27. A
28. C
29. C
30. B
31. B
32. C
33. B
34. B
35. B
36. C
37. C
38. B
39. B
40. A
41. A
42. B
43. A
44. C
45. A
46. C
47. C
48. B
49. B
50. A
51. B
52. B
53. B
54. C
55. A
56. A
57. B
58. C
59. B
60. A
61. C
62. A
63. A
64. C
65. C
66. B
67. C
68. A
69. B
70. B
71. C
72. A
73. B
74. A
75. B
76. B
77. C
78. C
79. B
80. A
81. C
82. C
83. B
84. B
85. B
86. C
87. A
88. B
89. B
90. B
91. A
92. B
93. A
94. A
95. C
96. A
97. C
98. B
99. C
100. B
101. A
102. A
103. B
104. B
105. A
106. A
107. B
108. C
109. B
110. A
111. B
112. C
113. B
114. A
115. B
116. A
117. B
118. A
119. B
120. C

Exam 2
Afternoon Session Answers

Answers referencing the Standards of Practice address Study Session 1, LOS 1.b, c and 2.a, b, c, except where noted.

1. **A** Expressing negative opinions about the CFA Program or CFA Institute is not a violation, according to guidance for Standard VII(A) Conduct as Members and Candidates in the CFA Program.

2. **A** To comply with GIPS, firms must list discontinued composites for at least five years after discontinuation. (Study Session 1, LOS 4.a)

3. **B** According to Standard II(B) Market Manipulation, members are prohibited from intentionally misleading market participants through the artificial manipulation of prices or trading data. Wilson's actions with regard to Bonner stock are not intended to mislead market participants but are related to a legitimate trading strategy and thus do not violate the Standards. Even though taking the short position may have played a part in moving the price of Bonner stock, it was not intended to manipulate the price. Wilson did, however, deceive market participants through his message board post related to Hatch stock. Thus, Wilson violated Standard II(B) in this situation.

4. **A** Standard I(A) Knowledge of the Law states that when applicable law and the Code and Standards have differing requirements, candidates and members must follow the strictest of the law where they reside, the law where they do business, or the Code and Standards.

5. **A** According to Standard V(B) Communication with Clients and Prospective Clients, clients must be made aware of the investment process used by the member and must be informed of any changes to this process. Additionally, members must include factors relevant to the analysis, determined using their reasonable judgment, in communications with clients. A change in the firm's valuation model is likely important information to clients. Green has informed all clients and prospects of the change in the model and has stated an expectation of improved results from the model without guaranteeing results or stating the improvement as fact. Smith has not violated the Standards.

6. **A** Stating that Baker passed the exams in consecutive years is acceptable, if in fact he did so, according to Standard VII(B) Reference to CFA Institute, the CFA Designation, and the CFA Program.

7. **A** Gifts from a client are distinguished from gifts from entities attempting to influence the portfolio manager's behavior, such as a broker. Deininger has complied with Standard I(B) Independence and Objectivity because he disclosed the gift from the client to his employer. This requirement is in place so that the employer can monitor the situation to guard against any favoritism towards the gift-giving client. The Standards do not require disclosing this gift to other clients. Permission would be required if the client's gift was to be based on future account performance.

8. C According to Standard VI(A) Disclosure of Conflicts, members and candidates must disclose to their clients, prospects, and employer all situations that could reasonably be expected to compromise their independence and objectivity. Stock ownership of a company in which clients are invested would need to be disclosed to clients and the employer since a member may be tempted to purchase more stock for client accounts in order to increase the value of personal holdings. Participation on the board of directors of a company in which clients are invested would also need to be disclosed to both clients and the employer. Board positions may inhibit the member's ability to objectively determine when to sell the stock of the company and may expose the member to material nonpublic information.

9. B According to Standard II(A), an analyst may not use material nonpublic information. The information is material to the company's future profitability, and is nonpublic because the lawsuit has not yet been filed and is not yet a matter of public record. The mosaic theory does not apply here, because the mosaic theory assumes that the nonpublic information gathered is nonmaterial.

10. A According to Standard III(A) Loyalty, Prudence, and Care, members must put client's interest ahead of their employer's or their own interests. Members have a duty of loyalty, prudence, and care. Also, members must comply with any applicable fiduciary duties in the client relationship. Welch has violated his duty of prudence by investing the Craig Family Trust assets in a manner inconsistent with the trust investment mandate which stated the trust should have a risk/return profile that mirrors the S&P 500 Index using a passive strategy. Welch also violated Standard III(C) Suitability by intentionally deviating from the investment policy statement. It is irrelevant that the strategy was successful.

11. B Rutherford is not treating all clients fairly and is thus violating Standard III(B) Fair Dealing. If he has an opinion regarding a possible surprise earnings announcement, he should include it in his published report.

12. B Under Standard III(C) Suitability, the investment advisor should consider the following in writing an investment policy statement (IPS) for each client: (1) client identification (type and nature of clients, existence of separate beneficiaries, and approximate portion of total client assets; (2) investment objectives (return objectives and risk tolerance); (3) investor constraints (liquidity needs, time horizon, tax considerations, legal and regulatory circumstances, unique needs and preferences); and (4) performance measurement benchmarks. Standard VI(A) Disclosure of Conflicts requires that members and candidates disclose all potential areas of conflict to clients, but this disclosure is not part of a client's IPS.

13. C Issuing a press release is the best way to achieve fair public dissemination. Notifying any specific analysts first is a violation of Standard III(B) Fair Dealing, regardless of any help they may have provided in the past.

14. C Standard II(B) Market Manipulation, is not intended to prohibit transactions that are done to minimize income taxes, or trading strategies that are not intended to distort prices or artificially inflate trading volume. Thus, neither Gordon nor Turpin is in violation.

15. A According to Standard V(A) Diligence and Reasonable Basis, group consensus is not required in the course of preparation of analytical reports. Pickler would only need to have her name removed from the report if she believed the investment committee did not have a reasonable and adequate basis for their changes.

16. **A** Under Standard VI(A) Disclosure of Conflicts, Malone is required to disclose to his employer all matters, including beneficial ownership of securities or other investments that reasonably could be expected to interfere with his duty to his employer or ability to make unbiased and objective recommendations. In addition, under Standard VI(A), Malone must disclose to clients all matters, including beneficial ownership of securities or other investments, that reasonably could be expected to impair his ability to make unbiased and objective recommendations. Members beneficially own securities or other investments that they or a member of their immediate family own or that are held in trust for them or their immediate family.

17. **C** Although Chavez was arrested, Standard I(D) Misconduct is not intended to cover acts of "civil disobedience." Standard IV(A) Loyalty, Chavez has a duty of loyalty to her employer. While she will not be compensated for the Greensleeves' Board position, the duties may be time-consuming and should be discussed with her employer in advance.

18. **B** Smith has violated Standard I(C) Misrepresentation by copying proprietary computerized information without authorization of the owner, Bright Star Bank and now Mega Bank. Even if Bright Star has been absorbed by Mega Bank, the assets of the trust department, including the model, now belong to Mega Bank, even if it chooses not to use them. Smith would have complied with the Standard if she had obtained permission from Mega Bank to copy the model.

19. **B** Because the Ivy Foundation has a minimum acceptable return that is greater than the risk-free rate, the safety-first ratio is a more suitable criterion than the Sharpe ratio for choosing the optimal portfolio. Given a set of available portfolios, the one that maximizes the safety-first ratio will minimize the probability that the return will be less than the minimum acceptable return if we assume returns are normally distributed. This is the optimal portfolio. Minimizing standard deviation of returns could lead to choosing a portfolio with an expected return below Ivy Foundation's minimum acceptable return. (Study Session 3, LOS 9.n)

20. **B** Since the median is higher than the mean, the distribution is negatively skewed. If the mean were higher than the median the distribution would be positively skewed. (Study Session 2, LOS 7.j,k,l)

21. **A** The conditional probability of recession given higher oil prices is 40%. The joint probability of recession and higher oil prices is determined using the multiplication rule for probability: $P(AB) = P(A \mid B)P(B)$. In this case, $P(A \mid B) = 0.40$ and $P(B) = 0.3$ (the probability of higher oil prices). The joint probability of higher oil prices and recession = $0.3 \times 0.4 = 0.12$. (Study Session 2, LOS 8.d,f)

22. **B** In a normal distribution, large deviations from the mean (in the "tails" of the distribution) are less likely than small deviations from the mean. A normal probability distribution is completely identified by its mean and standard deviation and has a mean equal to its mode and median. (Study Session 3, LOS 9.j)

23. **B** Because Investment 1 is compounded annually, its effective annual interest rate is equal to the stated annual rate of 6.1%.

Investment 2 has an effective annual interest rate equal to:

$[1 + (0.06 / 12)]^{12} - 1 = 6.17\%$

Investment 3 has an effective annual interest rate equal to:

$[1 + (0.059 / 4)]^{4} - 1 = 6.03\%$

Jones should choose Investment 2 since it has the highest effective annual interest rate. (Study Session 2, LOS 5.c)

24. **B** Relative class frequency for the class "0 up to 10" = 25 / 500 = 0.05. (Study Session 2, LOS 7.c)

25. **A** The *p*-value of a hypothesis test is the smallest significance level at which the null hypothesis can be rejected. Because both tests' *p*-values are less than 10%, both null hypotheses can be rejected at the 10% significance level (or at the 90% confidence level). One of the tests has a *p*-value greater than 5%, so the null hypothesis being tested cannot be rejected at the 5% significance (95% confidence) level. Neither test has a *p*-value less than 1%, so neither null hypothesis can be rejected at the 1% significance (99% confidence) level. (Study Session 3, LOS 11.e)

26. **A** The complete tree diagram is as follows:

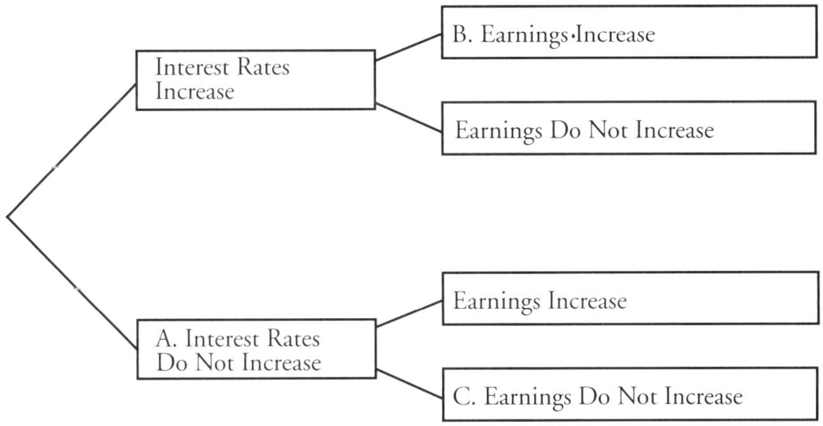

Cell A represents the unconditional probability that interest rates do not increase. Cell B represents the conditional probability that *earnings* increase, given that *interest rates* increase. Cell C represents the conditional probability that earnings *do not* increase, given that interest rates do not increase. (Study Session 2, LOS 8.j)

27. **A** The level of significance is the probability of rejecting the null hypothesis when it is true. The probability of rejecting the null when it is false is the power of a test. (Study Session 3, LOS 11.b)

28. **C** A random number generator is used to ensure that each member of the population has an equal chance of being selected. A sample in which each member has an equal chance of being selected is known as a simple random sample. In contrast, for stratified random samples, the population is split into mutually exclusive groups or strata, and simple random samples are extracted from each strata. In the example above, however, only one group is being sampled (growth stocks). So, Weaver is not correct. The distribution of a sample statistic, such as the sample mean, is known as a sampling distribution. Alternatively, the sampling distribution is the probability distribution of the sample means obtained from repeated sampling from the same population. The distribution of the sampled stocks is not the sampling distribution. Thus, Palmer also is incorrect. (Study Session 3, LOS 10.a)

29. **C** On a point-and-figure chart, the horizontal axis represents changes in the direction of the price trend. A technical analyst drawing a point-and-figure chart will fill squares in the same column until the price trend reverses, and then move to the next column. (Study Session 3, LOS 12.b)

30. **B** $-100{,}000$ = PV; 6 = N; $-100{,}000$ = PMT; 950,000 = FV; CPT → I/Y = 10%. (Study Session 2, LOS 5.e)

31. **B** Time-weighted returns are appropriate when the client exercises discretionary control over timing and amount of additions and withdrawals to the portfolio.

    Time-weighted $=[(1 + 0.15)(1 + (-0.05))]^{0.5} - 1 = 0.0452$ or 4.52%. (Study Session 2, LOS 6.d)

32. **C** Rao uses an ordinal scale. A nominal scale places data in groups but with no meaningful ranking content. An ordinal scale groups data according to a characteristic that can be ordered, such as grouping stocks based on their rates of return. Ratio scales are the strongest scale of measurement. Ratio scale amounts can be meaningfully added, subtracted, multiplied, and divided. Rao's ranking does not rise to this level (e.g., a group 4 firm does not necessarily have twice the interest coverage of a group 2 firm). (Study Session 2, LOS 7.a)

33. **B** The economic short run is the period in which a firm's plant size and technology are fixed. All factors of production can be changed in the long run. Input quantities of labor and raw materials can be changed in the short run. One year or the firm's operating cycle, whichever is longer, is the time frame typically used to distinguish between current and long-lived assets or liabilities on a balance sheet. (Study Session 4, LOS 15.h and Study Session 8, LOS 26.d)

34. **B** To get the inverse supply and demand functions, we must invert each function to get:

    $Q_S = P/0.05 - 0.84/0.05 = 20P - 16.8$

    $Q_D = 180(4) - (4)P = 720 - 4P$

    At a price of 30, $Q_S = 583.2$, $Q_D = 600$, and excess demand is approximately 17 units. (Study Session 4, LOS 13.f,g)

35. **B** While the central bank can control short-term interest rates, their relationship to long-term interest rates is not direct or proportionate. Long-term nominal interest rates include a premium for expected inflation. If a central bank's policy actions to reduce short-term rates cause market participants to expect higher future inflation, long-term rates will not decrease as much as short-term rates, and may actually increase.

    Open market operations by the central bank directly change the amount of bank excess reserves. Because various forms of short-term financing are close substitutes, the relationship among different short-term rates is closer than the relationship between short-term rates and long-term rates. (Study Session 5, LOS 19.j,m)

36. **C** When the Federal Reserve purchases Treasury securities in the open market, the supply of loanable funds increases and interest rates decrease, with the likely result of increasing economic growth. One of the Fed's intermediate targets is the federal funds rate that banks charge each other for loans. When the Fed conducts open market operations, it is generally to adjust the federal funds rate to its target level. The Fed cannot simply dictate the federal funds rate as it can the discount rate, so it must use open market operations to achieve its target. The purpose of using the federal funds rate is to achieve the Fed's primary goal of price level stability (or predictable inflation rates). In pursuing price level stability, the Fed also attempts to achieve its secondary goal of sustainable real GDP growth, which occurs when real GDP and potential GDP are close to each other. (Study Session 5, LOS 19.j)

37. **C** The consumer price index (CPI) is the average cost of a basket of goods and services, weighted to represent the purchases of a typical household, and indexed to a reference base period. The inflation rate is a percentage change in a price index such as the CPI. Inflation as measured by the CPI is believed to overestimate the actual increase in the cost of living because it does not account for structural changes such as new goods, quality improvements, or consumers shifting their purchases to lower-priced goods. (Study Session 5, LOS 18.f,g)

38. **B** When a market is subsidized by a government, the supply curve (marginal cost curve) shifts to the right while the demand curve (marginal benefit curve) stays constant. Producers in the market end up receiving more than the equilibrium price for their product and consumers in the market end up paying less than the equilibrium price for the product. In addition, the quantity produced and consumed is greater than the equilibrium quantity that would prevail without the subsidy. In this situation, the marginal cost of the product is greater than the marginal benefit, resulting in a deadweight loss due to overproduction and a surplus of the commodity. (Study Session 4, LOS 13.j,k)

39. **B** In the short run, real GDP can be less than its full-employment level (a recessionary gap that causes downward pressure on prices) or more than its full-employment level (an inflationary gap that causes upward pressure on prices). In long-run macroeconomic equilibrium, actual real GDP is equal to potential real GDP and there is no upward or downward pressure on the price level. (Study Session 5, LOS 17.i)

40. **A** The PAS/LDR cross rate is (1.70 BCS/LDR) / (3.2 BCS/PAS) = 0.5313 PAS/LDR. (Study Session 6, LOS 21.d)

41. **A** For all firms, profit is maximized at the output where the incremental revenue from selling an additional unit (marginal revenue) is equal to the incremental cost of producing it (marginal cost). Since marginal revenue is still higher than marginal cost, Tetra can expand output. (Study Session 4, LOS 15.g, 16.d)

42. **B** This is an example of monopolistic competition, because this market has low barriers to entry and exit, and features product differentiation. (Study Session 4, LOS 16.a,h)

43. A In this case, there are no clear potential benefits from trade because the countries' opportunity costs of production are equal. Colfax's opportunity cost of rice = 10 / 15 = 0.67 units of plastic, and Birklund's opportunity cost of rice = 12 / 18 = 0.67 units of plastic. Colfax's opportunity cost of plastic = 15 / 10 = 1.5 units of rice, and Birklund's opportunity cost of plastic = 18 / 12 = 1.5 units of rice. (Study Session 6, LOS 20.c)

44. C Gross domestic product (GDP) and gross national product (GNP) measure the value of final goods and services produced during the period. Gains from reselling assets purchased in an earlier period do not reflect current production and are not counted in GDP or GNP. The difference between GDP and GNP is that GDP measures output produced by factors of production located within the country, while GNP measures output produced by factors supplied by the country's citizens. (Study Session 5, LOS 17.d and Study Session 6, LOS 20.a)

45. A The proxy statement provides information about management and board member compensation, as well as any conflicts of interest. (Study Session 7, LOS 22.e)

46. C Strategic investments in companies are considered long term in nature and would likely not be converted into cash over the next year or less. (Study Session 7, LOS 23.a)

47. C The trademark is an intangible asset with an indefinite life, and its cost is not amortized. The decrease in the trademark's balance sheet value must be the result of impairment. For the intangible asset to appear on the balance sheet, Degen must have purchased the trademark. If Degen had developed the trademark internally, it would have expensed the cost rather than capitalizing it to the balance sheet. (Study Session 9, LOS 30.a,b,h)

48. **B** ROE = tax burden × interest burden × EBIT margin × asset turnover × financial leverage. The ratio of EBT to EBIT is the interest burden. Increasing financial leverage will increase a positive ROE. Decreasing the ratio of EBT to EBIT or decreasing asset turnover will decrease a positive ROE. (Study Session 8, LOS 28.d)

49. **B** Using accelerated depreciation for tax purposes while using straight line depreciation for financial reporting results in a deferred tax liability. In the United States, firms that use LIFO inventory accounting for financial statements must also use LIFO for tax reporting. Therefore, no deferred tax items can be associated with this accounting choice for GreenCo. Restructuring expenses generally result in a deferred tax asset (not a deferred tax liability) because the expense is not deducted for tax purposes until a later date. (Study Session 9, LOS 31.h)

50. A Restructuring and plant shutdown costs are considered part of a company's normal operations. Gains and losses related to discontinued operations are reported separately in the income statement because these activities are no longer included as part of the company's continuing operations. (Study Session 8, LOS 25.f)

51. **B** Deferred tax assets result from gains that are taxable before they are recognized in the income statement, while deferred tax liabilities result from gains that are recognized in the income statement before they are taxable. Deferred tax assets result from losses that are recognized in the income statement before they are tax deductible, while deferred tax liabilities result from losses that are tax deductible before they are recognized in the income statement. (Study Session 9, LOS 31.b)

52. **B** Diluted EPS is computed assuming conversion of the options using the treasury stock method. Accordingly, an additional 50,000 shares are added to compute diluted EPS: ($15 average market price – $10 exercise price) / $15 average market price × 150,000 options = 50,000 shares. 2,000,000 shares + 50,000 shares = 2,050,000 shares. (Study Session 8, LOS 25.g)

53. **B** The interest coverage ratio is EBIT / interest payments, and the fixed charge coverage ratio is (EBIT + lease payments) / (interest payments + lease payments). If EBIT and the interest coverage ratio are unchanged, interest payments are also unchanged. The decrease in the fixed charge coverage ratio must result from an increase in lease payments. Changes in working capital or financial leverage cannot be determined using only the information given. (Study Session 8, LOS 28.b,c)

54. **C** The unrealized loss on trading securities is reflected in net income. The total change in stockholder's equity is:

    $45,000,000 – [(1,000,000 + 500,000 shares) × $1.3/share] + (500,000 × $20/share) = $53,050,000

    (Study Session 8, LOS 26.f)

55. **A** According to U.S. GAAP, issuances of common stock and dividend payments are financing cash flows, and interest payments are operating cash flows. Depreciation is a non-cash operating expense. Acquisitions, divestitures, and investments in joint ventures are investing cash flows: –$175 million + $86 million – $50 million = –$139 million. (Study Session 8, LOS 27.a)

56. **A** Operating cash flow is equal to $36.1 million ($43.7 million net income + $4.2 million depreciation expense – $8 million gain on sale – $1.5 million increase in receivables – $2.3 million decrease in payables). Net capital expenditures are equal to $20 million ($35 million equipment purchased – $15 million proceeds from sale). Free cash flow to the firm is equal to $16.1 million ($36.1 million operating cash flow – $20 million net capital expenditures). (Study Session 8, LOS 27.i)

57. **B** The total cost of goods available for sale is $14,700 [(100 units × $15) + (200 units × $21) + (100 units × $18) + (300 units × $24)]. The average cost per unit is $21 ($14,700 / 700 units available for sale). Stanley sold 550 units (700 units available – 150 remaining). Thus, COGS is $11,550 (550 units sold × $21 per unit). (Study Session 9, LOS 29.c)

58. **C** An increase in the tax rate will increase the carrying values of both a deferred tax asset and a deferred tax liability. (Study Session 9, LOS 31.e)

59. **B** One of the general requirements stated in IAS No. 1 is that firms not offset assets against liabilities unless a specific standard permits or requires it. The statement of cash flows is not prepared using accrual accounting. IAS No. 1 states that firms should present comparative information for prior periods unless a specific standard states otherwise. (Study Session 7, LOS 24.e)

60. **A** Investing cash flows are most closely linked to a firm's noncurrent assets. Operating cash flows are most closely linked to a firm's current assets and current liabilities. Financing cash flows are most closely linked to a firm's noncurrent liabilities and equity. (Study Session 8, LOS 27.e)

61. **C** Since the asset's future undiscounted cash flows exceed its carrying value, no impairment is recognized. Thus, both ratios are correctly stated. (Study Session 9, LOS 30.h)

62. **A**

$$\text{Basic EPS} = \frac{\text{Net income} - \text{preferred dividends}}{\text{weighted average number of common shares outstanding}}$$

$$\text{Basic EPS} = \frac{830{,}000 - (6.5 \times 20{,}000)}{500{,}000} = 1.40$$

(Study Session 8, LOS 25.g)

63. **A** It is the coupon payment, not the interest expense, that results in an outflow of cash. The difference between the coupon payment and interest expense is the discount amortization. The amortization does not result in a cash outflow. Under U.S. GAAP, the coupon payment is reported as an operating cash flow. The discount, when paid at maturity, is reported as a financing cash flow. (Study Session 9, LOS 32.a,b)

64. **C** Commitments to outside parties to achieve aggressive results are identified in Statement of Auditing Standards No. 99 as a risk factor related to attitudes and rationalizations. Risks to the personal wealth of company managers are a factor related to incentives and pressures that may lead to fraud. Ineffective monitoring by management is a factor related to opportunities for fraud. (Study Session 10, LOS 33.c)

65. **C** As compared to an operating lease, a finance lease will result in higher interest expense. Thus, the interest coverage ratio is lower (higher denominator). A finance lease would add debt to the balance sheet, generating a *higher* debt-to-capital ratio. Because interest expense is higher in the early years of a finance lease, net income will be lower in the early years as compared to an operating lease. Over time, interest expense decreases as the liability is reduced through principal payments, resulting in higher net income in the later years of the lease. Thus, ROE will be lower in the early years (lower numerator) and higher in the later years (higher numerator). (Study Session 9, LOS 32.g,h,l)

66. **B** An auditor will issue a qualified opinion if the financial statements include exceptions to applicable accounting standards and will explain the nature and effect of these exceptions. An auditor will issue an adverse opinion if the financial statements are not presented fairly. (Study Session 7, LOS 22.d)

67. **C** Capitalizing the cost of the asset results in higher CFO and lower CFI in the period of the purchase, compared to expensing the entire cost. If the cost is expensed, the cash outflow is classified as CFO, but if the asset is capitalized, the cash outflow is classified as CFI. Cash flow from financing is not affected by the decision to capitalize. (Study Session 9, LOS 30.a)

68. **A** Completed contract is the appropriate revenue recognition method for long-term projects when revenue or costs cannot be estimated reliably. Under the completed contract method, no profit may be recognized until a project is completed, but an expected loss on a project must be recognized immediately. (Study Session 8, LOS 25.b)

69. **B** Several decision criteria are available when evaluating a standalone project. These criteria include net present value (NPV), profitability index (PI), and internal rate of return (IRR). The decision rules for these measures are as follows.

NPV:	If NPV > 0, accept project
	If NPV < 0, reject project
PI:	If PI > 1, accept project
	If PI < 1, reject project
IRR:	If IRR > required return, accept project
	If IRR < required return, reject project

(Study Session 11, LOS 36.d)

70. **B** Nonbank finance companies are a source of short-term financing for smaller firms and firms with lower credit ratings. Commercial paper issuance and revolving credit agreements are typically only available to larger corporations with high credit ratings. (Study Session 11, LOS 40.g)

71. **C** The four typical steps in the capital budgeting process are generating ideas, analyzing project proposals, creating the firm-wide capital budget, and monitoring decisions and conducting a post-audit. Raising additional capital is not one of the typical steps in the capital budgeting process. (Study Session 11, LOS 36.a)

72. **A** The formula for the asset beta is:

$$\beta_{asset} = \beta_{equity}\left[\frac{1}{1+\left(\frac{D(1-t)}{E}\right)}\right]$$

Therefore, the two betas are identical only if the company has no debt in its capital structure (D = 0). If the company has no debt, then the asset beta must equal the equity beta. (Study Session 11, LOS 37.i)

73. **B** Recall that the marginal cost of capital (MCC) is the cost of the last dollar of new capital raised by the firm. Marginal cost increases as increasing amounts of capital are raised during a set period. In general, firms in riskier businesses, or with riskier projects, have higher costs of common equity and thus higher MCC and WACC. The increase in the tax rate would reduce the after-tax cost of debt, reducing the MCC. (Study Session 11, LOS 37.a,b)

74. **A** Allowing shareowners to remove a board member is supportive of shareowner protection because shareowners can ensure that the board is comprised of individuals that represent shareowner interests. Staggered multiple-year terms for board members (a classified board) is not supportive of shareowner protection as it prevents shareholders from being able to change the board's composition if board members fail to represent shareowners' interests. Allowing the board to fill a vacant position for a remaining term is not supportive of shareowner protection, because it does not allow the shareowners to determine if the selected board member represents their interests. (Study Session 11, LOS 41.b)

75. **B** Nagle has no breakeven quantity of sales because the price per unit is less than Nagle's variable cost per unit (i.e., the contribution margin is negative). Nagle's operating income would be 900,000(\$3.25 – \$3.75) – \$400,000 = –\$850,000 by operating in the next period, but Nagle can limit its operating loss to its fixed operating costs of \$400,000 by shutting down temporarily. (Study Session 4, LOS 15.e and Study Session 11, LOS 38.d)

76. **B** The net operating cycle (also called the cash conversion cycle) measures the amount of time between paying the firm's suppliers for raw materials and collecting cash through the sale of finished goods.

$$\text{net operating cycle} = \frac{\text{number of days}}{\text{of inventory}} + \frac{\text{number of days}}{\text{of receivables}} - \frac{\text{number of days}}{\text{of payables}}$$

Gathers Company has decreased its net operating cycle, indicating it has decreased the number of days of inventory (more efficiently managed inventory purchases, processing, and fulfillment), decreased the number of days of receivables (reduced credit terms to customers and reduced collection times), or increased the number of days of payables (lengthened the amount of time to pay suppliers). The industry, however, has increased its average net operating cycle over the same period, indicating the industry has become less liquid by increasing number of days of inventory or number of days of receivables or decreasing number of days of payables. (Study Session 11, LOS 40.c)

77. **C** An investment policy for short-term portfolios should have the following elements: purpose, authorities, limitations/restrictions, quality, and other items. The purpose section should state the general reason the portfolio exists and the general strategy that will be followed. The authorities section should state the executives who will oversee the portfolio. The limitations section generally states the types of investments that are or are not acceptable and should note only categories of securities rather than specific issuers of securities (making answer choice C incorrect since it is too specific). The quality section should state guidelines for the credit quality of the investments in the portfolio. The "other" section may be used for portfolio requirements not covered in the first four sections, such as auditing or reporting requirements. (Study Session 11, LOS 40.e)

78. **C** Giving shareholders the ability to approve an external auditor allows them to evaluate the external auditor and express their opinion regarding whether the auditor serves their interests. The external auditor should report to the audit committee, not the firm's management, to avoid management influence. Audit committee members should be independent so that their interests are aligned with shareowners and not management. (Study Session 11, LOS 41.e)

79. **B** Investing on margin in the market portfolio will increase both risk and expected returns. This strategy would be mean-variance efficient. Other strategies such as shifting a portion of total funds to higher risk assets would achieve the higher return goal but would leave the portfolio below the CML and thus would not be an optimal strategy. (Study Session 12, LOS 44.a,b)

80. **A** Beta is equal to the covariance of the asset's returns with market returns divided by the variance of market returns. Beta can also be calculated as the *correlation* of the asset's returns with market returns multiplied by the ratio of the standard deviation of the asset's returns to the standard deviation of the market's returns. (Study Session 12, LOS 44.e)

81. C Risk averse investors prefer lower to higher risk for a given level of expected return and will only accept a riskier investment if they are compensated with higher expected return. A risk averse investor does not avoid all risk. (Study Session 12, LOS 43.d)

82. C Diversification reduces the portfolio standard deviation below the weighted average of the standard deviations if they are less than perfectly positively correlated. However, the minimum standard deviation occurs when the correlation is equal to negative one, not zero. (Study Session 12, LOS 43.e,f)

83. B For Royal Company, the required return equals 0.05 + 1.5(0.11 – 0.05) = 14%. The analyst predicts the stock will return 15%, implying that she thinks Royal Company stock is undervalued. (Study Session 12, LOS 44.h)

84. B When determining an investor's risk tolerance, an advisor should analyze the investor's personal situation, but should also gauge the investor's attitude toward risk. Risk tolerance is affected by the investor's psychological profile (i.e., willingness to take risk) as well as by the investor's ability to take risk. Age is an important influence on risk tolerance; younger investors generally are more able to withstand short-term losses because they have a longer time horizon in which to recover. Investors with high net worth are also more able to withstand short-term losses than investors with lower net worth, and thus tend to be more tolerant of risk. (Study Session 12, LOS 45.c,d)

85. B Apparel manufacturers are typically classified as consumer discretionary. Packaging firms are typically classified as basic materials and processing. (Study Session 14, LOS 50.b)

86. C The value effect refers to value stocks outperforming growth stocks on a risk-adjusted basis. Value stocks have low price-to-earnings or market-to-book ratios, or high dividend yields. Growth stocks have high price-to-earnings or market-to-book ratios, or low dividend yields. If the value effect persists over time and is not the result of inadequate adjustment for risk, buying value stocks will produce positive abnormal returns. (Study Session 13, LOS 48.f)

87. A The price-to-sales ratio can be used for firms with negative earnings and implicitly recognizes the value of assets not recognized on the balance sheet. The price-to-earnings ratio is the most popular ratio in the investment community; however, it is not a useful ratio for firms with negative earnings. One of the significant disadvantages of the price-to-book value ratio is that it does not recognize the value of nonphysical assets such as human capital or intangible assets generated internally. Therefore, price-to-book value would not be the best choice. (Study Session 14, LOS 51.h,k)

88. B New competitors are most likely to enter an industry during the growth stage of the industry life cycle. New entrants are less of a threat in the embryonic stage, when growth is slow and customer acceptance of the new product or service is highly uncertain. In the mature stage, the industry tends toward an oligopoly as competitors consolidate. (Study Session 14, LOS 50.h)

89. B Participating preference shares pay extra dividends if the firm's profits exceed a predetermined level. Convertible preference shares may be exchanged for the firm's common shares at a predetermined ratio. Cumulative preferred shares must be paid any omitted dividends from prior periods before the firm may pay dividends to common shareholders. (Study Session 14, LOS 49.a)

90. **B** Next year's dividend is $D_1 = D_0(1 + g) = \$1.90(1 + 0.06) = \$2.014$

Determine k_e using the CAPM: $RFR + \beta(R_{mkt} - RFR) = 5\% + 1.3(12\% \times 5\%) = 14.1\%$

Note that the market risk premium is $R_{mkt} - RFR$.

Calculate the stock's value using the infinite period dividend discount model (DDM):

$$V_0 = \frac{D_1}{k_e - g} = \frac{2.014}{0.141 - 0.06} = 24.86$$ (Study Session 14, LOS 51.e)

91. **A** Equity indexes typically require reconstitution only in response to corporate events, such as mergers or bankruptcies. Commodity indexes, which use futures contracts as their constituent securities, and fixed income indexes require frequent reconstitution as futures contracts expire and bonds mature. (Study Session 13, LOS 47.f,i,j)

92. **B** Using the derivative pricing rule, orders on an electronic crossing network are executed at fixed times of day at the average of the bid and ask quotes on the exchange where the security primarily trades. (Study Session 13, LOS 46.j)

93. **A** Net income = \$380 million × 12% = \$45.6 million

Cash flow = net income + depreciation & amortization = 45.6 + 44 = \$89.6 million

Cash flow per share = cash flow / number of shares = 89.6 million / 31 million = \$2.890

P/CF ratio = price / CF per share = 20.50 / 2.890 = 7.09. (Study Session 14, LOS 51.h)

94. **A** An order to buy if a price increases to a specified level is a stop buy order. A limit order at \$17 will execute immediately if the market price is \$15. A market order does not specify a price, but is executed at the prevailing market price. (Study Session 13, LOS 46.g,h)

95. **C** $D_1 = 1.5 \times 1.1 = 1.65$

$$\frac{P_0}{E_1} = \frac{\left(\frac{D_1}{E_1}\right)}{(k-g)} = \left(\frac{\frac{1.65}{4.70}}{(0.12-0.10)}\right) = \left(\frac{0.351}{0.02}\right) = 17.6$$

(Study Session 14, LOS 51.h)

96. **A** Because the yield on the preferred stock is less than its dividend rate, its price today is greater than its par value of \$1,000 and therefore must be greater than the price of any zero coupon bond with a face value of \$1,000.

The price of the preferred stock is \$58 / 0.054 = \$1,074.07.

The price of the zero coupon bond is $\$1{,}000 / [1 + (0.047 / 2)]^6 = \$869.91$.

(Study Session 14, LOS 51.d and Study Session 16, LOS 56.c)

97. **C** The analyst is correct with respect to bond maturity but incorrect with respect to coupon rate. As the maturity of a bond increases, an investor must wait longer for the eventual repayment of the bond principal. As the length of time until principal payment increases, the probability that interest rates will change increases. If interest rates increase, the present value of the final payment (which is the largest cash flow of the bond) decreases. At longer maturities, the present value decreases by greater amounts. Thus, interest rate risk increases as the maturity of the bond increases. As the coupon rate decreases, the interest rate risk of a bond increases. Lower coupons cause greater relative weight to be placed on the principal repayment. Because this cash flow occurs farther out in time, its present value is much more sensitive to changes in interest rates. As the coupon rate goes to zero (i.e., a zero-coupon bond), all of the bond's return relies on the return of principal which as stated before is highly sensitive to interest rate changes. (Study Session 15, LOS 53.c)

98. **B** The interest rate cap benefits the borrower who issues a floating rate bond. The cap places a restriction on how high the coupon rate can become during a rising interest rate environment. Therefore, the floating rate borrower is protected against ever-rising interest rates. (Study Session 15, LOS 52.e)

99. **C** The risk most likely to have increased is call risk, as the bonds have appreciated well above par value, quite possibly due to falling rates, which might motivate the issuer to call the bonds and replace them with lower cost debt. Credit risk has decreased, since the bonds have improved in rating from A to AA. There is no information to suggest that liquidity risk has changed, although a higher rated bond would likely be somewhat more liquid (less liquidity risk). (Study Session 15, LOS 53.a)

100. **B** "Tap system" refers to issuing bonds that are identical to a previous issue. (Study Session 15, LOS 54.a)

101. **A** For a bond with an embedded call option, the OAS is less than its zero-volatility spread by the option cost. Therefore, the zero-volatility spread is greater than the OAS for callable bonds. If the embedded call option has any value to the issuer, a callable bond with an OAS of 75 basis points will have a *Z*-spread that is greater than 75 basis points.

Because the OAS represents the bond's spread to the spot yield curve excluding the effect of the embedded option, it does not include any compensation for the volatility risk related to the option. The implied cost of an embedded option is the difference between the bond's zero-volatility spread (not the nominal spread) and its OAS. (Study Session 16, LOS 57.f)

102. **A** Bond Y will have the higher nominal spread due to the call option embedded in the bond. This option benefits the issuer, and investors will demand a higher yield to compensate for this feature. The option-adjusted spread removes the value of the option from the spread calculation, and would always be less than the nominal spread for a callable bond. Since Bond X is noncallable, the nominal spread and the OAS will be the same. (Study Session 15, LOS 55.g)

103. **B** First determine the arbitrage-free price of the bond by discounting the cash flows at their appropriate 6-month yields (i.e., one-half the BEY).

$$\frac{40}{1.037}+\frac{40}{1.035^2}+\frac{1,040}{1.0315^3}=1,023.50$$

The dealer can earn an arbitrage profit of \$4.00 by buying the bond for \$1,019.50 and selling the pieces for a total of \$1,023.50. (Study Session 16, LOS 56.f)

104. **B** If the yield curve is flat, the zero volatility spread is the same as the nominal spread. A steeper curve causes a greater difference between the spreads. An amortizing security (Bond Y) will exhibit greater difference in spreads than a non-amortizing one (Bond X). (Study Session 16, LOS 57.f)

105. **A** Putable bonds exhibit positive convexity at all yields. Callable bonds and mortgage passthroughs can exhibit negative convexity, defined as a decreasing sensitivity of the bond price to declining yields. Callable bonds and mortgage passthroughs exhibit less sensitivity to declining interest rates because both types of bonds provide the borrower a way out of high-cost debt as yields decline. The issuer of a callable bond tends to call the debt (at the stated redemption price, which is likely to be less than the market price of an otherwise identical non-callable bond) when interest rates decrease. The same explanation applies for mortgage passthroughs, attributable to the prepayment feature of mortgages (borrowers often refinance their mortgages as interest rates decrease, essentially ending the higher stream of cash flows flowing into the mortgage pool). (Study Session 16, LOS 58.c)

106. **A** Leverage and coverage ratios are data for analyzing company fundamentals, which is a step in the analysis of a firm's capacity to pay its debts. (Study Session 16, LOS 59.e)

107. **B** $(1+S_4)^4 = (1+{}_1f_0)(1+{}_1f_1)(1+{}_1f_2)(1+{}_1f_3)$

$(1.075)^4 = (1.06)(1.073)(1+{}_1f_2)(1.089)$

${}_1f_2 = 0.078$

(Study Session 16, LOS 57.g)

108. **C** This is an example of a negative covenant. Affirmative covenants are what the issuer must do (e.g., make timely payments of interest and principal, maintain equipment). A negative covenant refers to something the issuer is restricted from doing, such as paying dividends on stock when bond interest is in arrears. (Study Session 15, LOS 52.a)

109. **B** Original maturities are Treasury bills are less than 1 year, on Treasury notes from 2 to 10 years, and on Treasury bonds from 10 to 30 years. (Study Session 15, LOS 54.b)

110. **A** Inflation risk refers to the possibility that the purchasing power of a bond's future cash flows will be less than expected. Reinvestment risk is the possibility that the realized yield is less than the YTM because the bond's cash flows can only be reinvested at a rate less than the YTM. A bond with a price that responds more to an increase in interest rates than to an equal-sized decrease in interest rates is said to exhibit negative convexity. (Study Session 15, LOS 53.m)

111. **B** Losses on Carlson's portfolio of large cap stocks can be offset by gains on a short position in a futures contract. (Gains on the portfolio would be offset by futures losses.) He could also *buy* put options on the S&P 500. A long position in an S&P 500 forward contract would not offer any downside protection. (Study Session 17, LOS 60.c)

112. **C** Because Chen is short the futures contracts which are denominated in dollars per Swiss franc, an increase in the futures price means that Chen receives fewer dollars per franc sold than could a person contracting at the new price. Therefore her position decreases in value and the decrease is subtracted from her margin account. The reverse is true if the futures price decreases in value. Thus on the first day, the futures price increases by 0.9300 – 0.9120 = 0.0180. This is a loss of 100,000(0.0180) = \$1,800. At the end of the first day the margin balance is 4,000 – 1,800 = 2,200. Because the account balance is below the maintenance margin level, Chen would receive a margin call and would need to deposit enough to bring the account balance back to the initial margin level of \$4,000. Chen must deposit \$1,800. On the second day, the futures price falls and Chen realizes a margin account gain of 100,000(0.9300 – 0.8928) = \$3,720. The account balance at the end of the second day is 2,200 + 1,800 + 3,720 = \$7,720.

The following table summarizes the account balance changes.

Day	*Beginning Balance \$*	*Funds Deposited \$*	*Futures Price \$*	*Price Change \$*	*Gain/Loss \$*	*Ending Balance \$*
0	0	4,000	0.9120			4,000
1	4,000	0	0.9300	0.0180	(1,800)	2,200
2	2,200	1,800	0.8928	(0.0372)	3,720	7,720

(Study Session 17, LOS 62.d)

113. **B** A 3 × 6 FRA expires in 90 days (3 months from now) and is based on interest that will be paid 90 days after the expiration (6 months from now), which is 90-day LIBOR. (Study Session 17, LOS 61.f)

114. **A** The call writer's potential loss is unlimited, and the put buyer's loss exposure is limited to the \$3 premium paid. The put writer's potential gain is limited to the \$3 premium received, but the call buyer's potential gain is unlimited. The put writer's loss exposure is \$45 – \$3 = \$42 if the stock price declines to zero. (Study Session 17, LOS 65.a)

115. **B** European options can only be exercised at expiration. A put option gives the owner the right to sell the underlying asset. Put options are in-the-money when the strike price is above the underlying asset price. In this case, the option is in-the-money by \$35 – \$25 = \$10. (Study Session 17, LOS 63.b,c)

116. **A** The quarterly fixed rate payments on the swap are equal to \$200,000 [10,000,000 × (0.08 / 4)]. In exchange for this payment, Irczek will receive the return on the S&P 500 Index. If the return on the index is positive, the net payment Irczek must make will be lower than \$200,000, or may even be a cash inflow if the return on the index exceeds 2%. If the return on the index is negative, Irczek will have to make an additional payment on top of the fixed payment. Since Irczek owes \$400,000, the additional \$200,000 must result from a negative quarterly return on the index of \$10,000,000 / \$200,000 = 2%. (Study Session 17, LOS 64.b)

117. **B** Mezzanine financing in an LBO refers to the issue of securities that have both debt and equity features so that they are on the balance sheet between debt and equity. Mezzanine-stage financing refers to financing of different types that is employed during the period just prior to an IPO of a firm funded by venture capital. (Study Session 18, LOS 66.d)

118. **A** For financial reporting purposes the value of a position is calculated using either the average of the bid and ask or using the bid for *long* positions and the ask for *short* positions. In calculating the value of positions for trading purposes, funds often subtract a discount for illiquidity from accounting NAV, resulting in a lower trading NAV. (Study Session 18, LOS 66.e)

119. **B** Survivorship bias in hedge fund returns contributes to overstatement of performance and understatement of risk. (Study Session 18, LOS 66.c,g)

120. **C** A commodity market is contango if the futures price is higher than the spot price. (Study Session 18, LOS 67.a)

Exam 3
Morning Session Answers

To get valuable feedback on how your score compares to those of other Level I candidates, use your Username and Password to gain Online Access at schweser.com and choose the left-hand menu item "Practice Exams Vol. 2."

1. C	31. B	61. B	91. A
2. B	32. A	62. B	92. C
3. B	33. C	63. B	93. A
4. B	34. A	64. A	94. B
5. A	35. C	65. A	95. A
6. B	36. B	66. C	96. A
7. A	37. B	67. B	97. B
8. A	38. C	68. C	98. A
9. A	39. A	69. C	99. A
10. A	40. B	70. A	100. C
11. B	41. C	71. B	101. A
12. A	42. B	72. C	102. A
13. A	43. B	73. B	103. B
14. B	44. A	74. B	104. C
15. A	45. C	75. A	105. C
16. C	46. C	76. C	106. B
17. C	47. B	77. C	107. A
18. B	48. C	78. C	108. B
19. C	49. B	79. A	109. A
20. A	50. B	80. A	110. A
21. C	51. A	81. C	111. B
22. B	52. C	82. A	112. C
23. A	53. C	83. A	113. B
24. B	54. C	84. B	114. C
25. C	55. C	85. C	115. A
26. B	56. B	86. B	116. B
27. B	57. C	87. C	117. B
28. C	58. C	88. B	118. C
29. A	59. B	89. B	119. C
30. B	60. C	90. A	120. A

Exam 3
Morning Session Answers

Answers referencing the Standards of Practice address Study Session 1, LOS 1.b, c and 2.a, b, c, except where noted.

1. **C** Standard VII(B). According to the standard, members are not allowed to misrepresent or exaggerate the meaning of the CFA designation, membership in CFA Institute, or candidacy in the CFA program. This applies when the member references their relationship to the CFA Institute or CFA program verbally, or in writing (both print and electronic). Brown's statements regarding the Level III candidates at Brinton are acceptable. Stating that the analysts passed all three CFA exams on the first attempt is a statement of fact and is acceptable. Brown has also made acceptable statements regarding the rigor of the CFA program and has not over-promised investment results in connection with employing CFA charterholders and candidates. However, Brown's statement regarding the Level II CFA candidates at Brinton does violate Standard VII(A) by presuming that these Level II candidates will pass the next Level III exam and meet the work experience requirement.

2. **B** Bates plagiarized in violation of Standard I(C) Misrepresentation, because even though Bates might have eventually come to the same conclusion, he utilized other analyst's work and represented it as his own.

3. **B** It is likely that Johnson's outside work competes with her employer, especially since Smith Brothers caters to institutional clients. Standard IV(A) Loyalty requires that Johnson not engage in conduct that harms her employer. Permission from employer for the outside work is required.

4. **B** Standards I(B) Independence and Objectivity and V(A) Diligence and Reasonable Basis require the member to use reasonable care and judgment to achieve and maintain independence and objectivity in making investment recommendations or taking investment action. If Hanning believes the earnings projections do not have a reasonable basis, he should not permit the report to be issued under his name.

5. **A** Pollard has enough information to determine that the overheard information is indeed material nonpublic information. No matter how this information was obtained, even through an overheard conversation, Pollard may not act or cause others to act on it. Even if he had contacted internal counsel before placing the trade, Pollard would have violated Standard II(A) Material Nonpublic Information.

6. **B** Standard III(B) Fair Dealing. Members and candidates must deal fairly and objectively with all clients and should forgo any sales to themselves or their immediate families to free up additional shares of oversubscribed stock issues for clients. The fact that most clients will receive fewer shares than they requested is not a violation.

7. **A** According to Standard III(E) Preservation of Confidentiality, members and candidates must keep information about former, current, and potential future clients confidential unless client information is legally required to be disclosed, the information pertains to potential illegal client activities, or the client gives permission for the information to be disclosed. Crane is complying with current legal reporting requirements which require disclosure of personal client information for both former and current clients. Thus, Crane has not violated the Standard by disclosing the client information.

8. **A** Standard I(C) Misrepresentation does not prohibit members and candidates from making truthful statements that some investments, such as U.S. Treasury securities, are guaranteed in one way or another. Suitability does not become a concern until the potential clients take investment action.

9. **A** Brief presentations are acceptable if they include a statement that detailed information is available upon request. Standard III(D) Performance Presentation requires members and candidates to make reasonable efforts to ensure fair, accurate and complete presentation of results. While compliance with GIPS is recommended to meet Standard III(D) obligations, use of GIPS is not required.

10. **A** In accordance with Standard VI(B) Priority of Transactions, employer and client transactions must take priority over any personal transactions, meaning any transactions in which the member or candidate is the beneficial owner. Disclosure is not enough to comply with this Standard and the execution price is not relevant.

11. **B** Firms are encouraged, though not required, to have an independent third party verify GIPS compliance. (Study Session 1, LOS 3.c)

12. **A** Certain GIPS provisions apply to real estate investments. These provisions apply regardless of level of control the firm has over the management of the investment, and are unrelated to whether leverage is involved. (Study Session 1, LOS 4.d)

13. **A** Howell is using publicly available financial reports as well as non-material nonpublic information regarding the travel plans of the company's executive officers that led him to suspect that the company is planning a merger with a Japanese oil company. Thus, Howell formed his conclusion using the mosaic theory and did not violate Standard II(A) Material Nonpublic Information.

14. **B** Standard VI(A) Disclosure of Conflicts requires sell-side members or candidates to disclose beneficial ownership of securities they analyze. The Standard does not prohibit such beneficial ownership. For the purposes of compliance with Standard VI(A), beneficial ownership conveys the same obligations as owning the stock directly.

15. **A** Garcia has violated Standard IV(A) Loyalty because the records are the property of Peak Investments. Garcia may contact former clients but most obtain their contact information from public sources.

16. **C** GIPS requires that firms present, in their initial GIPS-compliant performance history, data for a minimum of five years or since the firm's inception. After the initial 5 years results are presented, the firm must add annual performance each year up to a minimum of 10 years. "Up to a minimum of 5 additional years" is incorrect because the initial GIPS-compliant presentation may not include 5 years of performance history (i.e., if "since inception" was a period less than 5 years). (Study Session 1, LOS 4.a)

17. **C** Members and candidates must identify the parties to whom fiduciary duty of loyalty is owed. In this case, Green's fiduciary duty is to the beneficiaries of the pension fund, not to Harris. If Green acts in Harris's best interests rather than the best interests of the beneficiaries, he will violate Standard III(A) Loyalty, Prudence, and Care.

18. **B** In accordance with Standard III(C) Suitability, a member or candidate acting as an investment advisor must make a reasonable inquiry into the client's objectives, constraints, and investment experience prior to making any investment recommendation. The Standard recommends preparing an Investment Policy Statement (IPS) for the client. Investments the client has made previously may be relevant to the client's investment experience, but Standard III(C) does not require the advisor to obtain specific information about which securities the client has previously invested in, although current holdings may be quite relevant.

19. **C** An empirical probability is established by analyzing past data. Note that the question is only asking about investors under the age of 30. In the survey, the number of investors under 30 was 325 + 235 = 560. The number of investors under 30 who did not make a stock trade was 325 / 560 = 0.58 or 58%. (Study Session 2, LOS 8.b)

20. **A** Phillips is interested in the probability of observing a result that is one standard deviation above the expected value for EPS. Approximately 68% of observations fall within plus or minus one standard deviation of the mean. Therefore, 1 – 0.68 = 0.32 or 32% remains in the tails. Since we are interested in the upper tail, we can say that there is 0.32 / 2 = 0.16 or 16% probability of observing an EPS greater than 3. (Study Session 3, LOS 9.m)

21. **C** The arithmetic mean is statistically the best estimate (expected value) of the next year's return. The harmonic mean is not typically used to compute the historical performance or forecast the expected performance of an investment; rather it is used to compute the average cost of shares purchased over time. The geometric mean is used to calculate average annual compound returns. It is the best estimate of future multi-year annual compound returns, but the arithmetic mean is the best estimate of a single year's return. (Study Session 2, LOS 7.e,m)

22. **B** The histogram contains a long left tail, which indicates significant negative skew for the distribution. If the histogram contained a long right tail, the distribution would have exhibited positive skew. A distribution with negative excess kurtosis (i.e., a platykurtic distribution) is less peaked and has thinner tails compared to a normal distribution. A distribution that is more peaked and has thicker tails compared to a normal distribution has positive excess kurtosis (i.e., a leptokurtic distribution). (Study Session 2, LOS 7.d,j)

23. **A** An opportunity cost is the amount foregone by pursuing a specific course of action. By holding onto cash, the individual is foregoing interest that could be earned by investing the cash. As interest rates rise, the opportunity cost of holding onto the cash also rises. Therefore, McGrow is correct. Interest rates are used to discount future cash flows in order to determine today's (present value) equivalent of the future cash flow amounts. The present value is inversely related to the discount rate. Therefore, Modello is also correct. (Study Session 2, LOS 5.a)

24. **B** Technical analysts believe the flow of information into the market is gradual, causing the market to adjust prices to a new equilibrium over a significant period of time. (Study Session 3, LOS 12.a)

25. **C** Because order is important, use the permutation formula to select 4 managers for a bonus out of the 7 managers eligible: 7! / (7 – 4)! = 7! / 3! = 5,040 / 6 = 840. (Study Session 2, LOS 8.o)

26. **B** This is a difference of means test where we want to know if the mean result of the new drug is greater than the mean result of the current treatment. The decision rule for the null hypothesis is H_0: $\mu_{New} - \mu_{Current} \leq 0$. Results from the new drug and the current treatment are likely to be independent, so a paired comparisons test is not appropriate. (Study Session 3, LOS 11.a)

27. **B** The 95% confidence interval is the range of possible stock returns that has 95% probability of including the hypothesized population mean. The decision rule is to not reject the null hypothesis if the hypothesized mean lies within the 95% confidence interval, and to reject the null hypothesis if the hypothesized mean lies outside the 95% confidence interval. The decision rule is to reject the null hypothesis whenever the (absolute value of the) calculated test statistic exceeds its critical value (i.e., the test statistic lies in the "rejection tail"). The power of a test is the probability of rejecting the null hypothesis when it is false. (Study Session 3, LOS 11.c)

28. **C** Gallant receives a €500 dividend on the MM preferred shares plus a €6,000 payment from Wood at the end of year 1. The preferred shares offer a perpetuity of €500, which Gallant sells at the end of year 1. At the end of year 1, the value (price received by Gallant) for the preferred stock equals €500/0.10 = €5,000.

$$\text{Holding period return} = \frac{5{,}000 + 6{,}000 + 500 - 10{,}000}{10{,}000} = 15\%.$$

(Study Session 2, LOS 6.c)

29. **A** Elliott wave theory defines an impulse wave as a wave in the direction of the prevailing trend. An impulse wave is composed of five smaller waves. A corrective wave (against the prevailing trend) is composed of three smaller waves. (Study Session 3, LOS 12.g)

30. **B** An ordinal scale puts data into categories that can be ordered with respect to some characteristic. A nominal scale places data into categories that have no particular order. In a ratio scale, data is ordered, differences in data values are meaningful, and ratios of values are meaningful. In this case, the securities are ranked in order with respect to buy/sell ratings, but the differences between ratings (e.g., the differences between 5 and 4 and between 4 and 3) are not necessarily uniform, and ratios of the ratings are not meaningful. (Study Session 2, LOS 7.a)

31. **B** According to the Central Limit Theorem, if the sample size is large, the sample mean will be distributed normally regardless of the population's distribution, specific inferences can be about the population mean, and the sample mean will have a standard deviation equal to the population standard deviation divided by the square root of the sample size (also known as the standard error). (Study Session 3, LOS 10.e)

32. **A** The major limitations of Monte Carlo simulation are that it is fairly complex and will provide answers that are no better than the assumptions used and that it cannot provide the insights that analytic methods can. Monte Carlo simulation is useful for performing "what if" scenarios. One of the first steps in Monte Carlo simulation is to specify the probably distribution along with the distribution parameters. The distribution specified does not have to be normal. (Study Session 3, LOS 9.q)

33. **C** For a price searcher firm, price discrimination can increase profits if the firm has two or more identifiable customer groups with different price elasticities of demand, and if customers who buy the product at a lower price cannot resell it to other customers. (Study Session 4, LOS 16.d)

34. **A** While under specific conditions a country that is a large importer of a good can increase its own economic welfare and that of other importing countries by imposing a tariff that decreases the world price of the good, imposing a tariff does not increase global economic welfare under any circumstances. For one or more countries to benefit from the imposition of a tariff, it must be the case that any net gains in economic welfare are offset by an even greater welfare loss in the exporting countries. (Study Session 6, LOS 20.e)

35. **C** Central banks control the growth of a country's money supply through their monetary policy actions. Many central banks also regulate their countries' banking systems and issue their countries' currencies. Fiscal policy (taxation and government spending) is generally the responsibility of a country's executive and legislative officials. (Study Session 5, LOS 19.a,f)

36. **B** Cost-push inflation is initiated by an increase in the price of a key productive input, which reduces short-run aggregate supply, decreasing real GDP to below its full-employment level (a recessionary gap), and increasing the price level. If the central bank responds by expanding the money supply, aggregate demand will increase, moving real GDP toward its full-employment level but increasing the price level further. If additional increases in input prices reduce SRAS and cause the central bank to further expand the money supply to restore full employment, cost-push inflation results. (Study Session 5, LOS 18.h)

37. **B** Collusion is an agreement among firms to avoid various competitive practices. The cartel practicing collusion will be similar to a monopoly, causing prices to increase and output to decrease compared to a competitive market. (Study Session 4, LOS 16.d)

38. **C** Factors that affect long-run aggregate supply (potential real GDP) include the quantity of labor available, the quantity of capital available, and the level of technology. An increase in aggregate hours worked is an increase in the quantity of labor, which increases long-run aggregate supply. An increase in expected inflation does not affect long-run aggregate supply, but causes aggregate demand to increase as consumers make purchases sooner and businesses increase investment in anticipation of higher profits. A decrease in the real wage rate increases short-run aggregate supply but does not affect long-run aggregate supply. (Study Session 5, LOS 17.h,l)

39. **A** The equation of exchange is MV = PY. If velocity (V) is increasing faster than real output (Y), inflation (P) would have to be increasing faster than the money supply (M) to keep the equation in balance. (Study Session 5, LOS 19.c,j)

40. **B** Neither statement is accurate. The minimum average variable cost will occur at a lower production level than the minimum average total cost. Profit is maximized where marginal revenue equals marginal cost, not where average total cost is minimized. (Study Session 4, LOS 15.d,g)

41. **C** The equilibrium price is 40:

$-120 + 5P = 440 - 9P; 14P = 560; P = 40$

At a price of 45, which is above the equilibrium price, quantity supplied is greater than the quantity demanded. Sellers will compete to offer the excess supply at lower prices until the price has decreased to its equilibrium level, reducing the quantity supplied and increasing the quantity demanded. (Study Session 4, LOS 13.d)

42. **B** Investing the domestic currency at the domestic interest rate should earn the same return as buying a foreign currency at the spot exchange rate, investing at the foreign interest rate, and selling the foreign currency proceeds at the forward exchange rate. If both currencies trade freely and participants can enter forward contracts, arbitrage trading will cause the percentage difference between the forward and spot exchange rates to be approximately equal to the difference between interest rates in the two countries. (Study Session 6, LOS 21.f)

43. **B** Economic profits are zero in the long run under monopolistic competition, but since average cost includes the costs of product differentiation and advertising (branding), there is disagreement over the efficiency of long-run output. Both advertising and product differentiation can create value as consumers prefer more choices and use the advertising and branding information to make purchase decisions. Whether there is an efficient amount of product differentiation or not, the benefits of product differentiation do tend to offset its costs. Whether the benefits of differentiated products totally offset the costs compared to a competitive market with a single (undifferentiated) product is open to debate. (Study Session 4, LOS 16.b)

44. **A** Marginal revenue is the change in total revenue per additional unit produced and sold. At a price of 18, quantity demanded is equal to 500 – 20(18) = 140, and total revenue is 140 × 18 = $2,520. At a price of 17.95, quantity demanded is equal to 500 – 20(17.95) = 141, and total revenue is 141 × 17.95 = $2,530.95. Marginal revenue for the 141st unit is 2,530.95 – 2,520 = $10.95. (Study Session 4, LOS 15.b)

45. **C** IFRS requires firms to use component depreciation. Each component of an asset is depreciated separately based on its estimated useful life. U.S. GAAP permits component depreciation but does not require firms to use it. (Study Session 9, LOS 30.c)

46. **C** Derivative instruments held by the firm are recognized at their fair market values on the balance sheet. Operating leases are a form of off-balance-sheet financing. Purchased brand names may be reflected in the value of intangible assets, but internally generated brand names do not appear as balance sheet assets. (Study Session 8, LOS 26.b,e)

47. **B** Asset turnover equals sales / average total assets. Understating depreciation expense has no effect on sales. The lower depreciation will result in understatement of accumulated depreciation, so assets will be overstated. The higher level of assets will decrease the asset turnover ratio. (Study Session 8, LOS 25.d, 28.b)

48. **C** Research expenses are ongoing costs of operations for a manufacturing firm. Losses or gains from the sale of a business segment are included in operating expenses. (Study Session 8, LOS 25.e,f)

49. **B** Basic EPS $= \dfrac{\$500\,\text{million} - \$20\,\text{million}}{100\,\text{million}} = \$4.80\,\text{per share}$

Preferred dividend = 5 million × \$4 = \$20 million

Shares created from conversion = 5 million shares × 3 shares = 15 million shares

$\dfrac{\$20\,\text{million}}{15\,\text{million}} = \$1.33$, convertible preferred is dilutive

Shares created from warrant $= \left[\dfrac{\$50 - \$25}{\$50}\right] \times 10\,\text{million shares} = 5\,\text{million shares}$

Exercise price < average price, warrants are dilutive.

Diluted EPS $= \dfrac{\$500\text{ million}}{100\text{ million} + 15\text{ million} + 5\text{ million}} = \$4.17$ per share

(Study Session 8, LOS 25.g)

50. **B** Management can boost reported earnings by increasing estimates of useful lives and salvage values for the company's depreciable assets. Both will increase reported earnings by reducing depreciation expense. Choices that increase reported earnings are generally considered to decrease the quality of reported earnings.

The cash flow earnings index is operating cash flow divided by net income. If this ratio is *less* than 1.0 consistently, the company is reporting higher earnings than are likely to be supportable by its operating performance. If the company is leasing an asset for only half the asset's useful life, an operating lease is likely appropriate. One of the criteria for a finance lease under U.S. GAAP is that the lease period is 75% or more of the asset's useful life. (Study Session 10, LOS 33.b,d)

51. **A** U.S. GAAP requires that goodwill associated with an acquisition be measured at the excess of the purchase price over the fair value of the acquired company's assets and recorded as an intangible asset. (Study Session 8, LOS 26.e)

52. **C** Unrealized gains and losses for trading securities are reported in the income statement, but unrealized gains and losses on available-for-sale securities are reported in other comprehensive income. Dividends and interest income from all the investments are included in pretax income. \$200,000 + 30,000 + 50,000 + 10,000 = \$290,000. (Study Session 8, LOS 26.e)

53. **C** Financial statement analysis refers to the use of information from a company's financial statements along with other information to make economic decisions regarding that company. Financial reporting refers to the reports and presentations that a company uses to show its financial performance to investors, creditors, and other interested parties. Financial reporting is a requirement for companies that are listed on public exchanges. (Study Session 7, LOS 22.a)

54. **C** Ignoring taxes, the cash flow for 20X1 consists of the sale proceeds. The sale proceeds equal \$35,000, or the \$20,000 book value (\$100,000 cost – \$80,000 accumulated depreciation) plus the \$15,000 gain. The proceeds are reported as an inflow from investing activities. (Study Session 8, LOS 27.a,f)

55. **C** FCFF = CFO + Int(1 − tax rate) − capital expenditures

$$FCFF = 3{,}500 + \left[195 \times \left(1 - \left(\frac{1{,}540}{4{,}400}\right)\right)\right] - 727 = 2{,}899.75 \approx 2{,}900$$

(Study Session 8, LOS 27.i)

56. **B** In a period of rising prices and rising inventory levels, FIFO results in the highest net income (lowest COGS). (Study Session 9, LOS 29.c)

57. **C** Analysts generally do not have access to the detailed information from which a company produces its financial statements. An analyst who suspects a company is using aggressive methods to increase revenues should examine the company's disclosures of accounting policies and compare these policies, along with the company's financial results and ratios, to those of similar companies. (Study Session 7, LOS 23.g, 24.i)

58. **C** Because an operating lease does not require that a liability be recognized on the balance sheet, as a finance lease does, the debt-to-equity and debt-to-assets ratios are lower if a lease is reported as an operating lease. Operating income is lower in the early years of an operating lease compared to a finance lease because the entire lease payment is considered an operating expense. The lease reporting method does not affect total cash flow, but it determines the extent to which the lease payments are classified as operating or financing cash flows. (Study Session 9, LOS 32.f,l)

59. **B** Since the carrying value of Cobra exceeds the fair value of Cobra, the goodwill is impaired. The implied fair value of goodwill is $500,000 ($5,000,000 fair value of Cobra – $4,500,000 net assets). The impairment loss is equal to $250,000 ($750,000 goodwill carrying value – $500,000 implied goodwill). (Study Session 9, LOS 30.h)

60. **C** Permanent differences, such as permanently reinvested earnings from an unconsolidated affiliate, cause the effective tax rate to be different than the statutory tax rate. Depreciation expense and warranty expense result in temporary differences, which create deferred tax liabilities and assets. (Study Session 9, LOS 31.i)

61. **B** An argument in favor of using the indirect method is that it links the income statement with the cash flow statement by focusing on the differences between net income and operating cash flow. Standard setting bodies permit either method but encourage use of the direct method. Companies that use the direct method must provide a disclosure that reconciles net income with cash flow from operations, similar information to what would be presented under the indirect method. (Study Session 8, LOS 27.d)

62. **B** Return on assets is 3.0 × 2.5 = 7.5% in Europe, 4.5 × 1.5 = 6.75% in Asia, and 1.5 × 4.0 = 6.0% in North America.

Assets are $200 million / 1.5 = $133.3 million in Asia, $500 million / 4.0 = $125 million in North America, and $300 million / 2.5 = $120 million in Europe.

Net income is 4.5% × $200 million = $9 million in Asia, 3.0% × $300 million = $9 million in Europe, and 1.5% × $500 million = $7.5 million in North America. (Study Session 8, LOS 28.e)

63. **B** Shelby's management will agree to the lending covenants to lower the interest rate on the credit facility. The existing bondholders and shareholders may have more risk since their respective interests are subordinate to the credit facility. (Study Session 9, LOS 32.d, and Study Session 15, LOS 52.a)

64. **A** Income tax expense = taxes payable + ΔDTL – ΔDTA. Income tax expense in 20X2 was 500 + (300 – 200) – (300 – 200) = 500. Income tax expense in 20X3 was 500 + (400 – 300) – (200 – 300) = 700. Income tax expense increased by 200. (Study Session 9, LOS 31.d)

65. **A** An extraordinary item is reported net of tax. At a 40% tax rate, the before tax loss was $20,000 [$12,000 extraordinary loss / (1 – 40% rate)]. When redeeming bonds, a loss occurs when the reacquisition price exceeds the carrying value. Thus, given the reacquisition price of $1,010,000 ($1,000,000 × 101%), the carrying value must have been $990,000 ($1,010,000 – $20,000). (Study Session 8, LOS 25.g, and Study Session 9, LOS 32.a,c)

66. **C** Both IFRS and U.S. GAAP require interest that accrues during the construction of a long-lived asset to be capitalized as part of the asset's cost, and not recognized as interest expense during the construction period. (Study Session 9, LOS 30.a)

67. **B** Since the quick ratio is greater than one, the percentage decrease in the denominator (current liabilities) is greater than the percentage decrease in the numerator (cash + accounts receivable + marketable securities). The denominator will decrease relatively more than the numerator. As a result, the quick ratio will increase. (Study Session 8, LOS 28.b)

68. **C** adjusted cost of goods sold Quip = 270,000 – (30,000 – 20,000) = 260,000

adjusted gross profit margin Quip = (350,000 – 260,000) / 350,000 = 0.257 ≈ 26%

(Study Session 10, LOS 35.e)

69. **C** Excess cash balances should be invested to earn a positive return, but should remain in liquid instruments with relatively stable values. Examples include U.S. Treasury bills, short-term federal agency securities, bank certificates of deposit, banker's acceptances, time deposits, repurchase agreements, commercial paper, money market mutual funds, and adjustable-rate preferred stock. (Study Session 11, LOS 40.d)

70. **A** For a board and its members to represent the interests of a firm's shareowners, it must possess the requisite skills and experience to make independent decisions. A board that lacks such skill and experience is likely to defer to management on key issues. Such behavior is detrimental to shareowners if management and shareowners' interests are different. Among the desirable qualities for a potential board member are prior board experience, significant stock ownership in the firm they will govern, necessary experience and qualifications, ability to make informed decisions about the firm's future, ability to act with care and competence, and regular board meeting attendance. A longstanding relationship with the firm's executives is not a desirable quality as the relationship may create undue loyalty to the firm's management rather than its shareowners. (Study Session 11, LOS 41.d)

71. **B** Banker's acceptances are guarantees from a bank on behalf of a firm that has ordered goods, stating that a payment will be made upon receipt of the goods. (Study Session 11, LOS 40.g)

72. **C** The NPV of Project A is higher than the NPV of Project B at any discount rate less than the crossover rate. Because Project A and Project B are mutually exclusive, we should select the project with the higher NPV. (Study Session 11, LOS 36.e)

73. **B** From the shareholders' viewpoint, their interests would be better served if the company hired a third party to conduct voting tabulation to ensure confidentiality and accuracy. The third party should also maintain the voting records.

    Requiring shareholder approval for proposed takeover defenses protects shareholders from management's refusal of a beneficial takeover. For example, if an acquirer offers twice the market value of Benson's common stock, shareholders can prevent Benson's managers from initiating a takeover defense.

    Having multiple classes of common shares is not in the interests of all shareholders if the voting rights of some classes of shares are separated from those shares' economic value. In this case, however, the voting rights and the economic claims on the company's assets of the Class 2 shares are proportional to those of the Class 1 shares (a Class 2 share is simply one-tenth of a Class 1 share). (Study Session 11, LOS 41.g)

74. **B** Externalities refer to the effects that the acceptance of a project may have on other firm cash flows. Cannibalization is one example of an externality. (Study Session 11, LOS 36.b)

75. **A** Paying cash to shareholders as dividends reduces current assets (cash) and shareholders' equity (retained earnings), which decreases liquidity ratios, such as the current ratio, quick ratio, and cash ratio, and increases leverage ratios, such as the debt-to-assets and debt-to-equity ratios. (Study Session 11, LOS 39.a)

76. **C** The quick ratio is defined as: (cash + marketable securities + accounts receivable)/ current liabilities. If current liabilities have remained constant, cash, marketable securities, or accounts receivable must have decreased. Inventory is not included in the quick ratio. (Study Session 11, LOS 40.b)

77. **C** The IRR is the discount rate that equates a project's initial cost with the present value of its future expected cash flows, i.e., for which a project's net present value equals zero. The correct IRR decision rule is to accept the project if IRR is greater than the required rate of return, and reject the project if IRR is less than the required rate of return. (Study Session 11, LOS 36.d)

78. **C** Before the repurchase, Walker's earnings yield = \$2 / \$50 = 4%. Because Walker's after-tax cost of debt is equal to its earnings yield, the share repurchase with borrowed funds will not change Walker's EPS. (Study Session 11, LOS 39.d)

79. **A** Risk averse investors prefer the lowest-risk investment for any given level of expected return, or the highest expected return for any given level of risk. A risk-averse investor might prefer a risky investment if she feels the expected return will be higher. (Study Session 12, LOS 43.d)

80. **A** The three major steps in the portfolio management process are planning, execution, and feedback. Asset allocation and security analysis are components of the execution step, as is portfolio construction. Preparation of an investment policy statement is a component of the planning step. Portfolio monitoring and rebalancing, as well as performance measurement and reporting, are part of the feedback step. (Study Session 12, LOS 42.c)

81. **C** Issues involving taxes fall in the tax concerns category, and issues regarding regulation fall in the legal and regulatory factors category. Specific guidance from the investor on permitted businesses for investment is included in unique needs and preferences. (Study Session 12, LOS 45.e)

82. **A** The return of the risk-free asset is certain, so its standard deviation will be zero and its covariance and correlation with other assets will be zero. Therefore, adding the risk-free asset to a risky portfolio will decrease the portfolio standard deviation. (Study Session 12, LOS 44.a)

83. **A** No calculations are needed. The real return is greater than the nominal return because the inflation rate is negative. The leveraged return is more negative than the nominal return because the investment lost value and leverage magnifies the loss. (Study Session 12, LOS 43.a)

84. **B** The capital asset pricing model is the equation for the security market line (SML): risk-free rate plus beta times market risk premium, where the market risk premium equals the difference between the expected market return and the risk-free rate. The starting point (intercept) for the SML is the risk-free rate (5%), and the slope for the SML is the market risk premium (8%). For Stock X, the required return equals 0.05 + 1.5(0.08) = 17%, and for Stock Y equals 0.05 + 2(0.08) = 21%. Linn predicts 20% for each stock. Therefore, Linn's predicted return for Stock X lies above the SML and for Stock Y lies below the SML. She should conclude that Stock X is undervalued and Stock Y is overvalued. (Study Session 12, LOS 44.h)

85. **C** This is a limit order. If the shares trade for €75 or below, Fontenot's broker will purchase the shares for him. If Fontenot had wanted to sell shares he already owned when the price dropped to €75.00, that would be a stop loss order. (Study Session 13, LOS 46.g,h)

86. **B** An operationally efficient market is a market in which the cost of each transaction is minimal. Informational efficiency means prices in the market reflect all information currently available to participants. Price continuity means that prices do not adjust much from one transaction to the next unless new information about firm value becomes available. (Study Session 13, LOS 46.k)

87. **C** Cumulative preferred shares stipulate that all preferred dividends must be paid before common stock dividends can be paid. (Study Session 14, LOS 49.a)

88. **B** Differences between the book value and market value of equity reflect investors' expectations about the amount and timing of a firm's future cash flows. Other things equal, repurchasing stock decreases both the book value and market value of equity, while neither a stock split nor a reverse stock split has any effect on the book value or market value of equity. (Study Session 14, LOS 49.g)

89. **B** D1 = 1.50

D2 = 3.00

D3 = 4.50

g = 0.06

required return = RFR + β(R_m – RFR)

required return = 0.02 + 1.3(0.08 – 0.02) = 0.098

$$P_3 = \frac{4.50 \times 1.06}{0.098 - 0.06} = \frac{4.77}{0.038} = 125.53$$

$$V = \frac{1.50}{1.098} + \frac{3.00}{(1.098)^2} + \frac{4.50 + 125.53}{(1.098)^3} = 102.08$$

(Study Session 14, LOS 51.e)

90. **A** In a short sale transaction, the lender of stock would not receive dividends from the issuing company. Therefore, if the company paid a dividend, the short seller would be required to pay that amount to the lender. The short seller must post some collateral or margin (usually the proceeds of selling the stock). (Study Session 13, LOS 46.e)

91. **A** Enterprise value equals the market value of a firm's common stock and debt minus its cash and short-term securities. Enterprise value is interpreted as the amount that would be needed to take over a firm. (Study Session 14, LOS 51.i)

92. **C** Diversification eliminates unsystematic risk, not systematic risk. The portfolio manager's duties require a thorough understanding of the client's current objectives and constraints. In addition, the portfolio manager must monitor them for any possible future changes. (Study Session 13, LOS 48.e)

93. **A** Private equity firms tend to be better able to focus on long-term performance than publicly traded firms because they do not face pressure from public shareholders to produce positive short-term results. Because their shares are not publicly traded, private equity firms are not required to comply with the same financial reporting regulations as publicly traded firms. As a result, private equity firms have lower compliance costs than comparable publicly traded firms, but less scrutiny from public shareholders may result in weaker corporate governance. (Study Session 14, LOS 49.c)

94. **B** Cost leadership is a competitive strategy in which a firm attempts to become the lowest-cost producer in the industry. This will enable the firm to offer lower prices than its competitors. A differentiation strategy involves making a product distinctive compared to competing products so that customers will be willing to pay a premium price. A competitive strategy is described as defensive if it is used to maintain a firm's market share and offensive if it is used to gain market share. (Study Session 14, LOS 50.k)

95. **A** Weighting countries in a multi-market index by market capitalization, rather than a fundamental factor such as GDP, is likely to overweight countries with previously high stock returns. (Study Session 13, LOS 47.h)

96. **A** The dividend payout ratio is 1 – expected retention ratio = 1 – 0.625 = 0.375 or 37.5%.

The leading (forward) P/E ratio is:

$$\frac{P_0}{E_1} = \frac{D_1 / E_1}{r - g} = \frac{0.375}{0.11 - 0.06} = 7.50$$

Multiplying the leading P/E ratio times forecasted earnings per share gives the stock value:

$P_0 = (P_0 / E_1)(E_1) = 7.50(\$4.24) = \$31.80$. (Study Session 14, LOS 51.h)

97. **B** The bond equivalent yield (BEY) is calculated by doubling the semiannual yield that, when compounded for two periods, would equal the annual yield. The BEY will always be less than the yield to maturity of an annual pay bond.

$\text{BEY} = 2 \times [(1.07)^{0.5} - 1] = 0.0688 = 6.88\%$

(Study Session 16, LOS 57.d)

98. **A** The liquidity preference theory states that investors require a liquidity premium for investing in longer-term bonds. This liquidity premium is compensation for interest rate risk and increases as maturities get longer. The liquidity preference theory can explain a flat or downward sloping term structure of interest rates as an expectation of decreasing future short-term interest rates. For the term structure to remain flat, according to this theory, the increasing liquidity premium must be accompanied by decreasing short-term interest rates so that the total interest rate (short-term rate + liquidity premium) is constant throughout time. A similar argument is made to justify a downward sloping term structure of interest rates. (Study Session 15, LOS 55.b,c)

99. **A** The implied rate on a repurchase agreement is generally less than the rate charged by banks for margin buying, especially when a service fee is added on to the margin interest rate by the broker. Margin percentage is regulated, but this restriction does not affect repurchase agreements. While in a repurchase agreement, the loan value is the value of the collateral reduced only by the implied interest (repo) rate. Repurchase agreements are much more common for institutional bond investors than margin buying. (Study Session 15, LOS 52.f)

100. **C** Neither coupon nor principal STRIPs have credit risk or reinvestment risk. They are direct obligations of the U.S. government that have no interim cash flows to be reinvested. There can be negative tax consequences, however, since the interest accrued each year is taxed even though no cash is received until the STRIP matures. (Study Session 15, LOS 54.c)

101. **A** Foreign currency debt ratings are typically lower than local currency debt ratings because the issuing government must acquire foreign currency to service that portion of its debt. Default risk is lower for local currency debt because the government can acquire local currency by collecting more taxes, reducing spending, or inflating the domestic money supply. (Study Session 16, LOS 59.j)

102. **A** The analyst is correct with respect to the redistribution of risk, but is incorrect with respect to total risk. Collateralized mortgage obligations (CMOs) were devised as a way of redistributing the prepayment risk of a mortgage backed security. In a CMO, the cash flows from the underlying assets are collected and distributed to different tranches according to a predetermined schedule. This reduces the uncertainty associated with prepayments for some tranches while increasing the uncertainty for other tranches. The total prepayment risk, however, is unchanged. (Study Session 15, LOS 54.f)

103. **B** The bond is trading at a premium, and if the bond is called at par that premium would be amortized over a shorter period, resulting in a lower return. The lower return is the more conservative number, so the YTC should be used. You could use your financial calculator to solve for YTC assuming 10 semiannual coupon payments of $35 (FV = 1,000; PMT = 35; PV = –1,065; N = 10; solve for i = 2.75; × 2 to get annual YTC = 5.5%). Calculation of YTM would use the same inputs except N = 20, to get YTM = 6.12% (Study Session 16, LOS 57.b)

104. **C** The conversion privilege is an option granted to the bondholder. The cap benefits the issuer. The accelerated sinking fund might reduce the investor's default risk, but the conversion option is the most likely benefit to the investor. (Study Session 15, LOS 52.e)

105. **C** For large portfolios, the full valuation approach requires that each bond be valued under each interest rate scenario. The duration/convexity approach would calculate the effect based on the overall portfolio characteristics, and would be much quicker. (Study Session 16, LOS 58.a)

106. **B** The value of the bond would increase due to the lower interest rates, but the increasing value of the option would offset some portion of this benefit. The value of the call option would increase, but this increase benefits the issuer, not the investor. (Study Session 15, LOS 53.b)

107. **A** Bond X carries the lowest investment grade rating. If it is downgraded, it will fall to a speculative rating, and many investors will be restricted from owning it. A downgrade would therefore have a more significant impact on Bond X. Bond Y carries a speculative rating that implies more risk of default than the higher rated Bond X. (Study Session 15, LOS 53.j and Study Session 16, LOS 59.a)

108. **B** Taxable equivalent yield = 0.045 / (1 – 0.35) = 0.0692 (Study Session 15, LOS 55.i)

109. **A** The yield on the bonds has increased, indicating that the value of the bonds has fallen below par. The bonds are therefore trading at a discount. If a bond is selling at a discount, the bond's current price is lower than its par value and the bond's YTM is higher than the coupon rate. Since Logan bought the bonds at par (coupon = YTM = 6%), the YTM has increased. (Study Session 15, LOS 53.b)

110. **A** LIBOR is the rate paid by banks borrowing from each other in the London Interbank market. The loan is made by way of a certificate of deposit (CD). The lending bank deposits funds into a CD account at the borrower bank. In this case, the CD would mature in six months. LIBOR can be denominated in several currencies, including the dollar, the pound, and the euro, but 6-month LIBOR is not the return on the shortest maturity euro-denominated instrument. LIBOR is not based on UK government security yields. (Study Session 15, LOS 55.j)

111. **B** Neither manager's statement is accurate. A covered call strategy generates income from the call premium but gives up the upside potential from an increase in the stock price. With a protective put strategy the upside potential is unlimited, but the maximum loss is equal to the stock price plus the put premium minus the exercise price of the put option. (Study Session 17, LOS 65.b)

112. **C** Statement 1 is correct. A futures contract is a standardized instrument that is traded on an exchange, unlike a forward contract which is a customized transaction. Statement 2 is incorrect. A forward contract is not marked to market. (Study Session 17, LOS 62.a,b)

113. **B** Quincy should enter into a long S&P 500 Index forward contract with Mason Inc. to minimize credit risk. Since the original short forward contract was with Mason Inc., entering into an offsetting position would allow for cancellation of the contracts between the two parties. Since Quincy is required to sell the underlying for $1,221, and the long contract has a price of $1,220, Quincy and Mason can terminate the original contract by having Mason pay Smith $1. Contracting with JonesCo or Redding Company would increase credit risk since Quincy would be exposed to potential default from another entity in addition to Mason. (Study Session 17, LOS 61.b)

114. **C** $C_0 \geq \text{Max}[0, S_0 - X / (1+ r)^{(219 / 365)}] = \text{Max}[0, 29 - 25 / 1.04^{0.6}] = \text{Max}[0, 29 - 24.42] = 4.58$. Note that this question can be answered without performing this calculation. Because the option is in the money by $4 and has time remaining until expiration, its minimum value must be greater than $4. Only choice C can be correct. (Study Session 17, LOS 63.k)

115. **A** At expiration, Kramer's call option on Blintz Company stock, Option 1, is in the money. The payoff on Option 1 is equal to $6 = ($64 – $58). The payoff occurs on the expiration day. A long position in a put option pays off when the underlying interest rate falls below the strike rate on the option. Since on the day of expiration LIBOR is 3.0%, Kramer's interest rate put option, Option 2, is in the money. The payoff on Option 2 is $6 = [$1,000 × (0.054 – 0.030) × 0.25]. However, the payoff occurs 90 days after the expiration date. Option 3 is out of the money. Therefore it has a payoff of zero. (Study Session 17, LOS 63.h)

116. **B** First, calculate the first fixed-rate payment as: $100,000,000 × [0.065 × (90 / 360)] = $1,625,000.

Next, calculate the first floating-rate payment as: $100,000,000 × [(0.052 + .01) × (90 / 360)] = $1,550,000

Since Anderson is paying fixed and receiving floating, the net payment from Anderson is $1,625,000 – $1,550,000 = $75,000 (a cash outflow). Notice you need only 90-day LIBOR since payments were being calculated quarterly and the question asked for the first net payment. (Study Session 17, LOS 64.b)

117. **B** Event-driven strategies attempt to capitalize on unique events or opportunities such as distressed debt or mergers and acquisitions. Relative value strategies involve taking long and short positions in related securities to exploit pricing inefficiencies. Macro strategy funds make directional trades on markets, currencies, interest rates, or other factors. (Study Session 18, LOS 66.d)

118. **C** The drawdown period for a private equity fund is the span of time over which the fund will draw down its committed capital and use it to invest in portfolio companies. Lockup periods and notice periods are related to hedge fund redemptions. (Study Session 18, LOS 66.d)

119. **C** Investment in commodities is most frequently implemented using futures contracts. One of the important motivations for investing in commodities is that they can serve as an inflation hedge. A commodity index strategy is considered an active strategy because commodity futures contracts expire and the manager needs to re-establish positions in long contracts and choose the margin collateral. Short-term securities posted as collateral must also be actively managed as they mature and need to be replaced. (Study Session 18, LOS 67.c)

120. **A** Investing in funds of funds is likely to result in lower returns net of fees over time compared to investing directly in hedge funds. Funds of funds receive net-of-fees returns from the funds in which they invest, and charge their own investors an additional layer of management and incentive fees. (Study Session 18, LOS 66.f)

Exam 3
Afternoon Session Answers

To get valuable feedback on how your score compares to those of other Level I candidates, use your Username and Password to gain Online Access at schweser.com and choose the left-hand menu item "Practice Exams Vol. 2."

1. A	31. C	61. A	91. B
2. B	32. B	62. B	92. A
3. B	33. C	63. C	93. A
4. C	34. C	64. C	94. A
5. A	35. B	65. B	95. B
6. A	36. B	66. A	96. B
7. C	37. B	67. B	97. A
8. A	38. A	68. C	98. A
9. C	39. A	69. C	99. A
10. C	40. A	70. C	100. B
11. A	41. B	71. B	101. A
12. B	42. B	72. C	102. C
13. A	43. B	73. A	103. A
14. C	44. B	74. B	104. B
15. C	45. C	75. C	105. B
16. C	46. A	76. B	106. C
17. B	47. C	77. B	107. A
18. A	48. A	78. C	108. C
19. B	49. B	79. B	109. B
20. A	50. C	80. A	110. C
21. B	51. A	81. B	111. A
22. C	52. C	82. A	112. A
23. C	53. C	83. B	113. A
24. A	54. C	84. B	114. C
25. C	55. C	85. B	115. B
26. C	56. B	86. B	116. C
27. C	57. A	87. C	117. C
28. B	58. A	88. B	118. B
29. B	59. A	89. B	119. B
30. A	60. A	90. A	120. B

Exam 3
Afternoon Session Answers

Answers referencing the Standards of Practice address Study Session 1, LOS 1.b, c and 2.a, b, c, except where noted.

1. **A** Brown has violated Standard I(C) Misrepresentation by giving prospects firm marketing materials that he knows are incorrect.

2. **B** GIPS-compliant results can be presented with non-compliant historical performance added for earlier periods, but no non-compliant results be presented for any time period after January 1, 2000. (Study Session 1, LOS 4.b)

3. **B** Although simultaneous distribution of information is preferred, distributing recommendations, or changes of recommendations, first to those clients who have previously expressed interest in these types of securities is acceptable. Giving preferred treatment to larger accounts would violate Standard III(B) Fair Dealing.

4. **C** Standard IV(B) Additional Compensation Arrangements requires Westerburg to obtain permission from his employer for any additional compensation from clients. He has done so. There is no requirement to notify other clients. Standard I(B) Independence and Objectivity distinguishes between gifts from clients and gifts from parties who may seek to influence a member's independent judgment and recommendations.

5. **A** According to Standard II(A) Material Nonpublic Information, an analyst may combine public information with nonmaterial nonpublic information (the mosaic theory). No additional disclosure is required.

6. **A** The exceptions are open-end or evergreen funds, which must follow regular GIPS. Other private equity investments should be valued in accordance with the GIPS Private Equity Valuation Principles. (Study Session 1, LOS 4.d)

7. **C** Kedzie has violated Standard I(C) Misrepresentation by guaranteeing that the return on ZYX stock will be positive.

8. **A** All of the statements are acceptable according to Standard VII(B), Reference to CFA Institute, the CFA designation, and the CFA Program. Koski is allowed to make a statement of fact such as the managers' right to use the CFA designation. Koski may reference the participation of his employees in the CFA program if the employees are currently registered to take one of the exams. The statements regarding dedication to the investment community and commitment to the highest ethical standards are proper references regarding the CFA program.

9. **C** All discretionary portfolios, whether closed or not, must be included in composite results for the period they were managed. Model results may not be included in composite results. (Study Session 1, LOS 3.b)

10. **C** Standard IV(A) Loyalty requires that members and candidates notify their employer all details of the independent practice and receive the employer's consent before engaging in the competitive activity, but does not require any statement from firm clients. If the independent practice is likely to affect clients negatively, the employer can refuse permission. Making preparations to begin a competitive practice is allowed, as long as it does not interfere with current employment duties.

11. **A** Standard II(A) Material Nonpublic Information states that if a member or candidate possesses material nonpublic information, they should make a reasonable attempt to have the information publicly disseminated, usually by encouraging the issuer company to inform the general public of the relevant information through a formal press release. Prohibiting all trading of ATI is not appropriate because it might give a signal to the market.

12. **B** According to Standard V(A) Diligence and Reasonable Basis, members must conduct professional activities in a diligent, independent, and thorough manner. If Manaugh chooses to update his report, it must be based on his own independent research and analysis, not an overheard conversation.

13. **A** Standard III(E) Preservation of Confidentiality states that members must maintain the confidentiality of all clients, prospects, and former clients unless the member has information concerning illegal activities, a disclosure of information is necessary by law, or the client grants permission to share the information. Members may share confidential client information with authorized employees who are also working for the client. Remy is allowed to inform Walker of the client's expected inheritance since Walker manages a portion of the client's portfolio and will likely need to prepare for the infusion of new funds into the account. Remy has also taken appropriate action by consulting with his firm's legal counsel about the possibility that the client's inheritance is part of an illegal scheme.

14. **C** Richards has violated Standard V(B) Communication with Clients and Prospective Clients by failing to appropriately distinguish between fact and opinion. It is her *opinion* that MegaRx will require a write-down, not a fact. Swanson violated Standard IV(C) Responsibilities of Supervisors by failing to recognize that the report he was personally reviewing contained a violation of the Code and Standards, which both he and Richards are bound to uphold.

15. **C** One of the firm's fundamental responsibilities under GIPS is to provide a compliant presentation to all prospects. Verification is not required. Firms are not permitted to alter historical composite performance because of changes in firm organization. (Study Session 1, LOS 4.a)

16. **C** Standard IV(C) Responsibilities of Supervisors requires members and candidates with supervisory responsibility to make reasonable efforts to detect and prevent violations of rules and regulations (as well as of the Code and Standards) by those under their supervision. The fact that violations occur is not necessarily evidence that reasonable efforts were not made. In large organizations, delegating supervisory responsibility may be necessary, but this does not relieve the person with overall authority of supervisory responsibility.

17. **B** Kevil has violated his duty under Standard III(A) Loyalty, Prudence, and Care. He must consider all proxy issues carefully and ensure that the proxies are voted in the best interest of his client. He cannot rely on the assumption that because a company's management happens to be the largest shareholders, they have his client's best interest in mind. He is allowed to use a more expensive broker for any client if the client specifically requests the use of the broker (client directed brokerage).

18. **A** Hoskins is attempting to manipulate the price of a derivative by securing a controlling position in the underlying asset, which is a violation of Standard II(B) Market Manipulation.

19. **B** The addition rule of probability is used to calculate the probability that at least one of two events will occur: P(A or B) = P(A) + P(B) – P(AB). The total probability rule is used to calculate the unconditional probability of an event given conditional probabilities related to the event: $P(A) = P(A|B_1)P(B_1) + P(A|B_2)P(B_2) + \ldots + P(A|B_N)P(B_N)$. The multiplication rule of probability is used to calculate the joint probability that two events will occur together: P(AB) = P(A|B) × P(B). (Study Session 2, LOS 8.e)

20. **A** A leptokurtic distribution (a distribution with kurtosis measure greater than 3) is more peaked in the middle (data more clustered around the mean) and has fatter tails at the extremes (greater chance of outliers). (Study Session 2, LOS 7.l)

21. **B** Chebyshev's inequality holds regardless of the shape of the distribution. For any k > 1, the minimum percentage of the distribution within k standard deviations of the mean is $1 - 1/k^2$. Thus, for 3 standard deviations, the percentage is $\geq 1 - 1/3^2 = 1 - 1/9 = 89\%$ (Study Session 2, LOS 7.h,l)

22. **C** Analyzing the ratio of stock prices to a stock index is known by technical analysts as relative strength analysis. (Study Session 3, LOS 12.b)

23. **C** The correlations for each pair of component securities are required to describe a distribution of returns for a portfolio. (Study Session 3, LOS 9.k)

24. **A** A discrete random variable is one that can be assigned at most a finite (countable) number of possible values (fractions or integers). (Study Session 3, LOS 9.b)

25. **C** The number of weighted portfolios is determined using the permutation formula:

$$_7P_4 = \frac{7!}{(7-4)!} = \frac{7!}{3!} = 840$$

The ordering of the 4 selected stocks matters because each stock receives an allocation that differs depending on its place in the ordering. For example, ABCD and ACBD are counted as two portfolios. (Study Session 2, LOS 8.o)

26. **C** Selecting only funds that managed to survive for 15 years should bias the value added upward, as poor-performing funds are more likely to have failed or been rolled into better performing funds (an example of survivorship bias). While the time period can affect results, with 15 years of data, the time period is likely to be less important than survivorship bias. (Study Session 3, LOS 10.k)

27. **C** Calculating the BEY is a two-step process. First, the HPY is converted to a semiannual effective yield. Second, the semiannual effective yield is multiplied by 2 to determine the BEY. The effective annual yield = $(1 + \text{HPY})^{365/90}$ and the money market yield = HPY × (360/90). (Study Session 2, LOS 6.f)

28. **B** Padgett's client is most concerned with getting less than a 4% return. Thus, the safety-first ratio is appropriate to measure risk. If the client was concerned about achieving a return less than the risk-free rate, the Sharpe ratio would be equivalent to the safety-first ratio. (Study Session 3, LOS 9.n)

29. **B** Hypothesis 1 is that "the mean 1-year Treasury bill rate should equal 4%." Therefore, the null hypothesis is: H_0: mean Treasury bill rate equals 4%; and the alternative hypothesis is H_a: mean Treasury bill rate does not equal 4%, which is a two-tailed test. Hypothesis 2 is that "the mean market risk premium should be positive." Therefore, the null hypothesis is: H_0: mean market risk premium is less than or equal to zero; and the alternative hypothesis is H_a: mean market risk premium is greater than zero, which is a one-tailed test. (Study Session 3, LOS 11.a)

30. **A** A consistent estimator is one that gets closer to the population parameter as the sample size increases. An unbiased estimator is one whose expected value equals the true population parameter. An efficient estimator has a variance of sampling distributions less than that of any other unbiased estimator of the population parameter. (Study Session 3, LOS 10.g)

31. **C** The interest rate equals the sum of the real rate, the expected inflation rate, the total risk premium (which equals the sum of the maturity risk premium, the liquidity risk premium, and the default risk premium). The real rate equals 1%, the expected inflation rate equals 2%, the maturity risk premium equals 4%. Treasury bonds have no liquidity or default risk, so the interest rate on a long-term Treasury bond would be expected to equal 7%. Since the SubPrime Providers (long-term) bond incurs default risk, its interest rate must exceed that of the long-term Treasury bond (i.e., 7%). The SubPrime Providers bond is highly liquid, so it has no liquidity premium. The default risk premium for SubPrime Providers bond equals 5%. Taken together, this implies that the SubPrime Provider bond interest rate should exceed the Treasury bond interest by 5 percentage points (12%). (Study Session 2, LOS 5.b)

32. **B** Bay is testing a hypothesis about the equality of variances of two normally distributed populations. The test statistic used to test this hypothesis is an *F*-statistic. A chi-square statistic is used to test a hypothesis about the variance of a single population. A *t*-statistic is used to test hypotheses concerning a population mean, the differences between means of two populations, or the mean of differences between paired observations from two populations. (Study Session 3, LOS 11.i)

33. **C** Diseconomies of scale are present when long-run average cost increases as output increases. The minimum efficient scale is the plant size that produces the quantity of output for which LRAC is at a minimum. (Study Session 4, LOS 15.f)

34. **C** There is a market equilibrium at a price of 250 and quantity of 750. The supply curve is downward sloping and intersects the demand curve from below; that is, the downward slope of the supply curve (–1/5) is less than the slope of the demand curve (–1/3). The equilibrium is unstable because there is excess demand above the equilibrium price and excess supply below the equilibrium price, either of which forces the price away from equilibrium rather than toward it. (Study Session 4, LOS 13.e)

35. **B** Central bank sales of securities reduce excess reserves in the banking system, causing interbank lending rates and other short-term interest rates to increase. If the monetary policy transmission mechanism operates normally, long-term interest rates should also increase, the domestic currency should appreciate, and economic growth and inflation should decrease. (Study Session 5, LOS 19.j)

36. **B** Since the labor force is the sum of employed and unemployed, a decrease in the labor force with the number employed held constant will decrease the unemployment rate (the number of unemployed divided by the labor force). The labor force participation rate is the labor force divided by the working-age population. If the labor force decreases while the working-age population remains the same, the participation rate will decrease. (Study Session 5, LOS 18.d)

37. **B** The absorption approach to analyzing how to improve a trade deficit suggests that in the absence of excess capacity in the economy, currency devaluation provides only a temporary improvement in a country's trade deficit that will reverse after the decrease in real domestic wealth from the currency depreciation is restored. It also concludes that a long-term improvement in the trade deficit requires either an improvement in the fiscal deficit or an increase in the excess of domestic savings over domestic investment. (Study Session 5, LOS 17.e, and Study Session 6, LOS 21.i)

38. **A** For a normal good, both the income and substitution effects are positive (i.e., they tend to increase consumption of the good). (Study Session 4, LOS 14.e)

39. **A** The slope of a consumer's budget constraint is equal to $-P_X / P_Y$. The original slope is $-8 / 20 = -0.4$, and the slope after the price decreases is $-6 / 14 = -0.429$. The absolute value of the slope increases (i.e., the budget constraint becomes more steeply sloped). (Study Session 4, LOS 14.c)

40. **A** Applying the Nash equilibrium model, Oil Tool will make the best possible decision based on Jones's potential decisions and Jones will make the best possible decision based on Oil Tool's potential decisions. If Oil Tool complies, then it must depend on Jones to comply, but complying is not in the interest of Jones. If Jones were to comply, then it must depend on Oil Tool to comply, but complying is also not in the best interest of Oil Tool. Both Oil Tool and Jones will conclude that the best course of action is to cheat on the pricing agreement. (Study Session 4, LOS 16.d)

41. **B** The Keynesian school of macroeconomics believes that increasing the money supply or increasing government spending (such as with a stimulus package) will increase real GDP and combat recession. Monetarists believe economic growth is best supported through a policy of steady and predictable money supply increases. The neoclassical school of thought believes that economic cycles will correct themselves through a rapid adjustment of the prices of key productive inputs that restores the economy to full employment. (Study Session 5, LOS 18.c)

42. **B** The real exchange rate is calculated as 0.75 BDE/TOL × 110/105 = 0.79 BDE/TOL. (Study Session 6, LOS 21.a)

43. **B** The quantity theory focuses on the quantity of money. The quantity theory states that velocity is not affected by monetary policy. Increasing banks' excess reserves would most likely lead to higher inflation. (Study Session 5, LOS 19.c)

44. **B** If price elasticity of supply is greater than price elasticity of demand, the impact on the price (net of tax) received by producers will be less than the impact on the price paid by consumers. As a result, consumers will pay a larger share of the tax. The actual incidence of a tax is unaffected by its statutory incidence, but it is affected by the relative elasticity of supply and demand for the good being taxed. (Study Session 4, LOS 13.j,k)

45. **C** Effects of inflation are likely to be discussed in management's commentary. For U.S. firms, inflation effects are among the items required to be addressed in Management's Discussion and Analysis. (Study Session 7, LOS 22.c)

46. **A** Classified balance sheets have categories for current assets, non-current assets, current liabilities, and non-current liabilities. (Study Session 8, LOS 26.c)

47. **C** Value stocks are described as having low price valuation ratios (price-book, price-cash flow, price-earnings, etc.). Using equity screens often results in under- or over-representation of certain industries in portfolios. Low price-to-book screens often result in an inordinate proportion of financial services companies. Growth stocks are described by above-average earnings growth rates. (Study Session 10, LOS 35.d)

48. **A** The FIFO method recognizes the oldest costs in the cost of goods sold. With rising prices, COGS will be lower and net income will be higher using FIFO as compared to the LIFO or average cost methods. Higher net income relative to sales (which are not affected by the inventory cost method) means higher profit margins. (Study Session 8, LOS 25.d)

49. **B** To qualify as an extraordinary loss, the loss must be both unusual and infrequent. The plane crash would most likely meet these criteria as it is unusual and would not be expected to recur. The other items would be unlikely to be considered unusual and infrequent. (Study Session 8, LOS 25.e)

50. **C** The stock split is applied retroactively to the beginning of the year. Since the preferred stock is not convertible, it has no impact on the number of common shares for calculating diluted EPS. Beginning shares (40,000 shares × 12 months) + split shares (40,000 shares × 12 months) – reacquired shares (20,000 shares × 6 months) = 840,000, and 840,000 / 12 months = 70,000 shares. (Study Session 8, LOS 25.g)

51. **A** Because all items on a common-size balance sheet are stated as a percentage of the same value (typically total assets), the quick ratio can be calculated from the given percentages: (30% – 10%) / 25% = 0.8. Neither the defensive interval nor working capital turnover can be determined using only the data given. (Study Session 8, LOS 26.h, 28.b)

52. **C** The trading portfolio classification includes the unrealized gain from the bond portfolio in net income, which is then recorded in retained earnings. Unrealized gains on available-for-sale securities are reported as other comprehensive income for the period and are recorded in accumulated other comprehensive income within owner's equity. Unrealized gains on held-to-maturity securities are not reported on the financial statements. (Study Session 8, LOS 26.e)

53. **C** Under IFRS, interest and dividends received may be shown as either cash flow from operations or cash flow from investing. Remember that in most cases, international standards are more flexible in reporting cash flow. (Study Session 8, LOS 27.c)

54. **C** Cash flow from operating activities is equal to $27.0 million [$120 million cash collected from customers – $96.5 million cash expenses + $3.5 million dividends received]. Depreciation expense is a noncash item. Acquiring an interest in an affiliate is an investing cash flow. Dividends paid and proceeds from reselling the company's own stock are financing cash flows. (Study Session 8, LOS 27.a)

55. **C** Revaluing the asset to £600,000 will increase future depreciation expense, and therefore reduce net income in subsequent periods. Because Vasco has not previously recognized a loss on this asset, the revaluation is not recognized as income but is recorded as an adjustment to equity. An increase in equity (with unchanged debt) will decrease the debt-to-equity ratio. (Study Session 9, LOS 30.g)

56. **B** When the replacement cost is between net realizable value and net realizable value less a normal profit margin, then market value is defined as replacement cost. When original cost is greater than replacement cost, under LCM, inventory is reported at replacement cost. (Study Session 9, LOS 29.f)

57. **A** Vertical common-size analysis of an income statement is typically done by stating each item as a percentage of sales. Stating each item on a financial statement as a percentage of its value in a base period is referred to as horizontal common-size analysis. (Study Session 8, LOS 28.a)

58. **A** Both of these judgments will result in the firm capitalizing expenses that had previously been expensed as incurred, increasing income as a result. Under IFRS, research costs are expensed as incurred but development costs are capitalized. Software development costs are expensed as incurred until technological feasibility is established, and capitalized after that point. (Study Session 9, LOS 30.a,b)

59. **A** The increase in equity that would be shown on the 20X9 statement of shareholders' equity would be $4 million, as common stock increased by $2 million and retained earnings increased by $2 million. Note that the years are displayed from right-to-left.

    The statement of cash flows for 20X9 would show a positive net cash flow of $10 million because the cash account on the balance sheet increased from $30 million to $40 million. Cash from financing will include a positive cash flow of $2 million related to issuance of common stock because the common stock account on the balance sheet increased from $39 million to $41 million. (Study Session 7, LOS 23.e)

60. **A** Low inventory turnover and declining revenue growth may be a sign that a firm has obsolete or slow-moving inventory. High turnover and low revenue growth may indicate too little inventory, while high turnover and high revenue growth may indicate efficient inventory management. (Study Session 9, LOS 29.h)

61. **A** The valuation allowance decreased from $11,700 to $8,100. The most likely explanation is the future earnings are expected to increase, thereby increasing the portion of the DTA that is likely to be realized. (Study Session 9, LOS 31.g)

62. **B** Service costs, which are the additional benefits that employees have earned during the period, are recognized as an expense on the current period income statement under both IFRS and U.S. GAAP. (Study Session 9, LOS 32.k)

63. **C** Use of more than one inventory cost flow method is permitted, but the same method must be used for items of a similar nature and use. (Study Session 9, LOS 29.b)

64. **C** Under both IFRS and U.S. GAAP, unrealized gains and losses on available for sale securities are recorded as other comprehensive income. LIFO inventory valuation is permitted under U.S. GAAP but not under IFRS. Interest received must be classified as an operating cash flow under U.S. GAAP, but may be classified as an operating or investing cash flow under IFRS. (Study Session 8, LOS 25.d, 26.e, 27.c)

65. **B** ROE = profit margin × total asset turnover × financial leverage. A decrease in financial leverage will result in a decrease in ROE. An increase in the profit margin will increase ROE. A loss reported in other comprehensive income will decrease shareholders' equity but not affect net income, which will increase ROE. (Study Session 8, LOS 25.k, 28.d)

66. **A** When a long-lived asset is sold or otherwise disposed of, its original cost and accumulated depreciation are removed from the balance sheet. Changing the estimated salvage value or useful life of a long-lived asset will change depreciation expense in the subsequent periods but does not affect accumulated depreciation. (Study Session 9, LOS 30.i,j)

67. **B** Tax depreciation is 200 / 4 = $50; book depreciation is 200 / 5 = $40. Thus, after two years, the carrying value is $120 [200 – (40 × 2 years)], and the tax base is $100 [200 – (50 × 2 years)]. The effective tax rate is not affected by temporary differences. The deferred tax *liability* at the end of the second year is $8 [(120 carrying value – 100 tax base) × 40%]. (Study Session 9, LOS 31.c)

68. **C** Stretching accounts payable (increasing days sales in payables) will increase operating cash flow. (Study Session 10, LOS 34.a)

69. **C** At points on the investment opportunity schedule that are above the marginal cost of capital curve, projects have higher IRRs than the cost of capital and these projects should be accepted. The amount of the optimal capital budget is at the intersection of a firm's investment opportunity schedule and its marginal cost of capital curve. Capital project investment up to this point creates firm value and increases shareholder wealth. Capital project investment beyond this amount would mean accepting projects with IRRs less than the marginal cost of capital. (Study Session 11, LOS 37.d)

70. **C** The yield to maturity correctly measures the pretax cost of debt financing. (Study Session 11, LOS 37.f)

71. **B** When the IRR and NPV methods conflict, the general rule is to take the higher NPV project, as NPV measures the expected increase in the value of the firm from undertaking the project. IRR is not the best measure for ranking mutually exclusive projects of different sizes, and the capital budget is not large enough to do both projects. (Study Session 11, LOS 36.d,e)

72. **C** The percentage change in EBIT caused by a 1% change in sales is the degree of operating leverage (DOL). The percentage change in EPS caused by a 1% change in sales is the degree of total leverage (DTL). Samor's DOL and DTL both equal 1.5. A degree of operating leverage greater than one results from fixed operating costs. Because DTL = DOL × DFL, Samor's degree of financial leverage must be equal to 1, which means Samor does not use debt financing. (Study Session 11, LOS 38.b)

73. **A** The operating cycle is days of inventory plus days of receivables. The cash conversion cycle is the operating cycle minus days of payables. Therefore, average days of payables are the operating cycle minus the cash conversion cycle. Dunhill's average days of payables (140 – 125 = 15) are less than Pierce's average days of payables (150 – 120 = 30). Which company has higher average days of inventory or receivables cannot be determined from the information provided. (Study Session 11, LOS 40.c)

74. **B** The analyst should use the target capital structure weighting if possible (i.e., if the firm has stated its target weights). If the targets are unknown, the analyst must estimate the weights. (Study Session 11, LOS 37.c)

75. **C** Sunk costs should be excluded from cash flows, as they are costs that cannot be avoided even if the project is not undertaken. Externalities, such as positive or negative effects of accepting a project on sales of the company's existing products, should be included in the cash flows. (Study Session 11, LOS 36.b)

76. **B** The correct method to account for flotation costs is to make the adjustment in the initial project cost. Adjusting the WACC is incorrect because flotation costs are a cash outflow at the initiation of the project, rather than an ongoing expense. Flotation costs can be substantial, typically 2% to 7% of the amount raised. (Study Session 11, LOS 37.l)

77. **B** The percentage of receivables outstanding for 31 to 60 days increased from 12% to 24%, while the percentage outstanding for 0 to 30 days decreased from 70% to 60%. Slower customer payments after the change in credit terms may indicate liquidity problems. (Study Session 11, LOS 40.f)

78. **C** GRE Financial's Board should be made up of a majority of independent board members to maintain its unbiased viewpoint. Takeover defenses, such as a poison pill provision, typically reduce shareholder value and should be viewed as a negative. (Study Session 11, LOS 41.b,c,g)

79. **B** The diversification ratio is the standard deviation of an equally weighted portfolio's returns divided by the average standard deviation of returns of the securities in the portfolio. Adding a security with a standard deviation equal to the average will decrease the portfolio standard deviation as long as the added security's returns are not perfectly positively correlated with the portfolio's returns. The result is a lower diversification ratio, which indicates a greater benefit from diversification. (Study Session 12, LOS 42.a)

80. **A** The SML uses either the covariance between assets and the market or beta as the measure of risk. Beta is the covariance of a stock with the market divided by the variance of the market. Securities that plot above the SML are undervalued and securities that plot below the SML are overvalued. (Study Session 12, LOS 44.f,h)

81. **B** Without a risk-free asset, an investor's optimal portfolio will be at the point where the investor's highest attainable indifference curve is tangent to the efficient frontier. Investors with different levels of risk aversion will therefore have different optimal portfolios. Johnson's optimal portfolio with have a lower expected return than Colson because Johnson is more risk averse than Colson, and his highest attainable indifference curve will be tangent to the efficient frontier at a lower expected return. (Study Session 12, LOS 43.d)

82. **A** Multi-factor returns generating models most often use fundamental and macroeconomic factors. Statistical factors have no basis in finance theory and are suspect as being the result of data mining, making them inappropriate risk factors in a multi-factor model. (Study Session 12, LOS 44.d)

83. **B** The efficient frontier represents the set of portfolios that has the highest expected return for a given level of risk. An indifference curve (in modern portfolio theory) represents the risk and return combinations that yield the same level of utility for an investor. An investor's utility curve (in modern portfolio theory) measures an investor's utility as a function of risk and return. (Study Session 12, LOS 43.g)

84. **B** Tactical asset allocation is deviating from a portfolio's strategic asset allocation because an asset class or sector is perceived to be mispriced in the short term. Establishing and updating target weights for asset classes based on the investor's objectives and constraints is strategic asset allocation. (Study Session 12, LOS 45.f,g)

85. **B** Margin call price =

$$P_0\left(\frac{1-\text{initial margin\%}}{1-\text{maintenance margin\%}}\right)=\$60\left(\frac{1-0.40}{1-0.20}\right)=\$60(0.75)=\$45$$

(Study Session 13, LOS 46.f)

86. **B** An important drawback of the price to book value ratio is that book values do not necessarily reflect market values. Book values of assets reported at amortized cost can be too low if prices have increased since the company acquired the assets. Book values can also be too high, for example, if technological changes have made some of a company's assets obsolete. The price to book value ratio is useful for valuing companies that primarily hold financial assets and for valuing companies that are expected to cease operations. (Study Session 14, LOS 51.k)

87. **C** The shakeout stage of the industry life cycle is characterized by slowing industry growth and profitability due to strong competition and overcapacity, with firms attempting to establish brand loyalty among their customers. In the mature stage of the life cycle, a smaller number of firms typically have strong brand loyalty. In the decline stage, capacity declines as firms exit the industry. (Study Session 14, LOS 50.h)

88. **B** Under cumulative voting, with three board seats up for election, the shareholder can cast up to 3,000 votes for one candidate. In a statutory voting system, an investor who holds 1,000 shares can cast 1,000 votes in the election for each seat. (Study Session 14, LOS 49.b)

89. **B** The semistrong form of EMH states that security prices rapidly adjust to reflect all publicly available information. If the analyst can use his model, which is based on publicly available information, to earn above average returns, the semistrong form of the EMH has been violated. If the semistrong form of EMH is violated, the strong form of EMH is also violated. (Study Session 13, LOS 48.d,e)

90. **A** Because the intrinsic value is more than the price, the investor should buy the stock. The required return is calculated using the following formula:

$$E(R) = RFR + \beta(R_M - RFR) = 0.04 + 1.25(0.08 - 0.04) = 0.09$$

Because the intrinsic value (30) exceeds the price (28), King should purchase the shares. Furthermore, because intrinsic value exceeds price, the expected return is above 0.09. With an expected return greater than the required return, King should buy Nacho Inc. stock. (Study Session 14, LOS 51.a)

91. **B** Calculate the dividends during the supernormal growth period using g_s = 15%.

$D_1 = D_0(1 + g_s) = \$2.00(1.15) = \$2.30$

$D_2 = D_0(1 + g_s)^2 = \$2.00(1.15)^2 = \$2.645$

$D_3 = D_0(1 + g_s)^3 = \$2.00(1.15)^3 = \$3.042$

D_3 is the first dividend that *will grow* at a constant rate. Use this dividend to calculate the value of the stock at t = 2 using the infinite period DDM.

$$P_2 = \frac{D_3}{(k_e - g)} = \frac{3.042}{0.12 - 0.07} = 60.84$$

Calculate the present value of the cash flows discounted at k_e of 12%.

PV of D_1 = \$2.30 / (1.12) = \$2.054

PV of D_2 = \$2.645 / $(1.12)^2$ = \$2.109

PV of P_2 = \$60.84 / $(1.12)^2$ = <u>\$48.50</u>

V_s = \$52.664 (Study Session 14, LOS 51.e)

92. **A** Trades in a call market occur at specified times. All orders are accumulated, and a single negotiated price is set that clears the market. (Study Session 13, LOS 46.j)

93. **A** It is difficult to price individual bond issues in an index because continuous trade data may not exist for some bonds. In addition, it is challenging to create a bond market index because the bond universe is much broader, and the price volatility of a bond (i.e., its duration) changes over time as the bond approaches maturity. (Study Session 13, LOS 47.i)

94. **A** The return on equity = profit margin × asset turnover × financial leverage

ROE = 10% × 0.75 × 1.6 = 12.0%

The retention rate = 1 – payout rate = 100% – 60% = 40%

g = (Retention rate) × (Return on equity) = 40% × 12.0% = 4.8%

(Study Session 14, LOS 51.e)

95. **B** An increase in the required rate of return would decrease the P/E ratio. An increase in the other two (the dividend payout rate and the growth rate) would increase the P/E ratio. This can be seen by inspecting the equation for the expected (P_0/E_1) ratio, which is:

$$\frac{P_0}{E_1} = \frac{D_1/E_1}{k - g}$$

where:
D_1/E_1 = the expected dividend payout ratio.
k = the required rate of return on the stock.
g = the expected constant growth rate of dividends.

(Study Session 14, LOS 51.h)

96. **B** The primary capital market refers to the sale of newly issued securities. Most issues are distributed through an underwriter, who handles the origination, bears the risk, and distributes the offering. A specialist is a dealer who represents an NYSE specialist firm. A specialist firm is one of the main facilitators of trade in existing securities on the exchange. Existing securities are traded in the secondary capital markets. (Study Session 13, LOS 46.i)

97. **A** The yield ratio is 8.75% / 5.25% = 1.67. The absolute yield spread is 8.75% – 5.25%, which is 3.50% or 350 basis points. The relative yield spread is 3.5% / 5.25% = 0.67 = 67%. (Study Session 15, LOS 55.e)

98. **A** Most CDOs are structured with senior and subordinated tranches. Securities that can be included in a CDO pool are not limited to those that are publicly traded (for example, bank loans can be in a CDO pool). Some CDOs (balance sheet CDOs) are sponsored by banks or insurance companies that seek to move the assets off their balance sheets, but others (arbitrage CDOs) are created by issuers that seek to earn a spread between the return on the assets and the rate promised on the CDO. (Study Session 15, LOS 54.j)

99. **A** The observed yield curve is upward sloping despite stable short-term rates. The pure expectations theory would predict a flat yield curve. The market segmentation theory can explain any shape of the yield curve, depending on supply and demand conditions for each time horizon. (Study Session 15, LOS 55.c)

100. **B** Clean price is the price excluding accrued interest, given as 976.25. The dirty price would add the accrued interest to get 976.25 + 14.92 = 991.17. (Study Session 15, LOS 54.c)

101. **A** Slowing economic growth reduces firm profitability and creditworthiness and causes yield spreads to widen. Higher-than-normal supply of new bonds can cause yield spreads to widen. Yield spreads tend to narrow during expansions when GDP growth rates are high. (Study Session 16, LOS 59.h)

102. **C** All else equal, a zero coupon bond has less reinvestment risk and more interest rate risk (duration) than a coupon paying bond. (Study Session 15, LOS 53.a)

103. **A** The distinction between effective convexity and modified convexity is that effective convexity accounts for the effects of embedded options on the bond's cash flows at different yields. For bonds that do not have embedded options, there is no difference between effective convexity and modified convexity. Both measures are used to improve the estimate of the change in a bond's price for a given change in yield. (Study Session 16, LOS 58.i)

104. **B** Yield volatility is positively related to the value of the embedded call option and negatively related to the value of a callable bond. The value of a callable bond is equal to the value of an option-free bond less the value of the call option. An increase in yield volatility will increase the value of the call option, decreasing the value of the bond. (Study Session 15, LOS 53.n)

105. **B** The prices of both bonds will converge to par value at maturity. (Study Session 16, LOS 56.d)

106. **C** The option cost is the difference between the zero volatility spread and the OAS, or 150 – 75 = 75 bp. With a flat yield curve, the nominal spread and zero volatility spread will be the same. (Study Session 16, LOS 57.f)

107. **A** The yield to maturity calculation assumes that all interim cash flows are reinvested at the yield to maturity (YTM). Since Horn's reinvestment rate is 7.5%, he would realize a return higher than the 7.0% YTM of the Kano bonds, or a return less than the 8.0% YTM of the Samuel bonds. (Study Session 16, LOS 57.c)

108. **C** The cap on these bonds is 8.5%, which would be reached when the 6-month Treasury yield reached 6.5%. The interest rate risk of floating rate bonds will be lower if the reset period is shorter, so an annual reset would mean higher risk than these bonds. Once a floating rate security hits its maximum (cap) rate, it will be priced similar to fixed rate bonds, since the ability of the coupon reset to keep pace with higher rates will be lost. (Study Session 15, LOS 53.e)

109. **B** Portfolio duration is the weighted average of component securities, using market values:

(2,400,000 / 7,200,000) × 4.625 + (3,600,000 / 7,200,000) × 7.322 + (1,200,000 / 7,200,000) × 9.3 = 6.753. (Study Session 16, LOS 58.g)

110. **C** The TIPS coupon rate is fixed. The coupon amount adjusts for inflation because the par value is periodically adjusted for inflation. The coupon rate is the real rate because it is the rate that the TIPS investor receives above the inflation rate. (Study Session 15, LOS 54.b)

111. **A** Forward contracts are private transactions in an unregulated market and the terms can be customized. However, forward contracts do have higher default risk as there is no clearinghouse to guarantee the performance of each party. Since the company is unwilling to accept credit risk from the counterparty, swaps and forwards will not be appropriate. (Study Session 17, LOS 60.c)

112. **A** The key advantages of derivatives markets are providing price information, reducing transactions costs, and shifting risks among market participants. Derivatives markets are highly efficient and arbitrage opportunities rarely exist or are quickly eliminated. (Study Session 17, LOS 60.d)

113. **A** The risk in writing a call is if the stock price increases. The premium is his maximum gain, but his potential loss is unlimited since the stock could have an infinite increase in value. (Study Session 17, LOS 65.a)

114. **C** The minimum value of an American put option is Max(0, X – S_0). Thus the lower bound for the put options on KCE stock is Max(0, 55 – 51.13) = $3.87. (Study Session 17, LOS 63.k)

115. **B** \$10M[(0.055 – 0.0475)(90 / 360)] / [1 + 0.055(90 / 360)] = \$10M(0.001875 / 1.01375) = \$18,496. (Study Session 17, LOS 61.g)

116. **C** $C = S + P - \left[X \Big/ (1 + RFR)^{T} \right]$

$$C = 33 + 2.75 - \left[30 \Big/ (1 + 0.055)^{\frac{80}{365}} \right] = 6.1$$

(Study Session 17, LOS 63.m)

117. **C** An existing single-family home for residential purposes will most likely be valued using the sales comparison method. (Study Session 18, LOS 66.e)

118. **B** Commodity ETFs are suitable for investors who are limited to buying equity shares. ETFs can invest in commodities or commodity futures and can track commodity prices or indexes. Buying shares of commodity-linked firms is less effective for gaining commodity price exposure because these share prices may not be highly correlated with commodity prices. Managed futures funds may not be available to an investor who is restricted to equity shares. (Study Session 18, LOS 66.d)

119. **B** Because poorer performing, less stable hedge funds are more likely to fail, survivorship bias causes returns to be overstated and risk to be understated in hedge fund databases. (Study Session 18, LOS 66.c,g)

120. **B** Returns on private equity investments depend to a large extent on the skill of the general partners. Private equity investments are illiquid and require a long-term investment horizon. (Study Session 18, LOS 66.d,e)

Notes

Notes

Notes

Notes

Notes

Notes

Notes

Notes

Notes